NO WONDER YOU FEEL LIKE CRAP!

NO WONDER YOU FEEL LIKE CRAP!

*The hidden, deadly connection
between stress, diet, and disease*

Richard Weinstein, D.C.

NO WONDER YOU FEEL LIKE CRAP!

copyright © 2013 by Richard A. Weinstein, DC
Cover design by Janice Hardy

All Rights Reserved, including the right to reproduce this book, or portions thereof, in any form whatsoever.

Neither the publisher nor the author of this book is engaged in rendering professional advice or services to the individual reader. The concepts, theories, procedures, and advice contained in this book are not intended as a substitute for a consultation with your physician. All matters regarding health issues require medical advice and supervision. Neither the author nor the publisher shall be liable or responsible for any loss, injury, or damage allegedly arising from any information or suggestion in this book, however caused. The opinions expressed in this book represent the personal views of the author and not necessarily those of the publisher.

While the author has made every effort to provide accurate telephone numbers and Internet addresses (URLs) at the time of publication, neither the publisher nor the author assumes any responsibility for errors or for changes that occur after publication.

Published by Richard A. Weinstein
523 Capitola Ave., Capitola, CA 95010
www.richardweinsteindc.com

ISBN: 978-0-692-36316-4

Second edition - January 2015

Printed in the U.S.A.

*For Lois, my dearest friend, my beloved wife,
and the finest person I have ever known*

ACKNOWLEDGMENTS

This book is the result of more than three decades of clinical experience and a continuous process of staying abreast of current research on hormonal function and imbalances, and learning how to resolve them.

There are two groups of wonderful people to thank in making this book a reality: those who mentored me to become a better doctor and taught me the pieces of the hormone physiological puzzle, and those who enabled me to write and publish this book.

First and foremost, my heartfelt thanks to Harry O. Eidenier, Jr., Ph.D., who gave me the initial insight into how to make sense of the incredible complexities of the human hormone system, and who has generously lent his time, support, and profound wisdom to this project. My thanks to David R. Seaman, D.C., who is a visionary regarding the destructive impact of inflammation on human health. I'm also deeply thankful to Datis Kharrazian, D.C., MneuroSci (and too many other degrees to list), for his incredible seminars that have enabled me and many other doctors to understand and keep pace with the research and therapeutic approaches for hormone and immune imbalances. Anyone who either studies or writes about the subject of stress owes an enormous debt of gratitude to Robert M. Sapolsky, Ph.D. A researcher at Stanford University, Dr. Sapolsky is by any standards, a genius in the field of human stress physiology, a wonderful and often hilarious writer, and a terrific human being. I want to thank Jack MacDonald, owner of the 41st Avenue Vitamin Center in Capitola California, for allowing me to use his vast knowledge of vitamin and nutritional supplements to help my patients.

A big hug and thanks to Dario Ciriello, who did the initial editing of my book, who kept me focused and on track, and who always believed in the value of this project. He has also been an inspiration in my revising the material and making it easier to understand.

Last, writing a book is a very time-consuming enterprise, and it can be a challenge if you already have a full-time job, as I do with my practice. None of this would have been possible without the support of my wife, Lois, and her tireless efforts to pick up the slack in managing my office and our home while I sat at the computer, writing. Clearly, I have a lot of lawns to mow and dishes to wash to make up for all of this, and I'm forever grateful for her loving support.

CONTENTS

Preface

1 THE JOURNEY BEGINS
A Chiropractor's Odyssey with Stress

7 THE CORTISOL PARADOX
The Stress and Inflammation Hormone

19 PHYSICAL STRESS AND THE PRO-INFLAMMATORY DIET
There's a Fire Down Below

38 TESTING CORTISOL LEVELS
The Conditions for Murder Are Met

42 THE RELATIONSHIP OF CORTISOL TO OTHER DISEASES
The Missing Link

69 RESOLVING CORTISOL IMBALANCES
A Plan That's Easy to Follow and Swallow

91 MAKE THE PAIN GO AWAY
Treating Causes Instead of Symptoms

112 THE NOT-SO-COMMON COMMONSENSE DIET
You're Actually Going to Put That in Your Mouth?

143   PSYCHOLOGICAL STRESS
"It's all in your mind, you know." —George Harrison

156   THE EMOTIONAL COMPONENT
OF ILLNESS
*A Tricky Roadblock on the Way to
Regaining Good Health*

172   CONCLUSION

Appendices

174   Handy Reference: A review of the 3R program

177   Glossary

189   Resource Guide

191   References

206   About the Author

PREFACE

When I began writing the original text of this book, then titled *The Stress Effect*, ten years ago, no-one other than an endocrinologist (hormonal specialist) or a hormone researcher would have been familiar with the adrenal hormone, *cortisol*.

The central theme of this book, as well as the single most important thing you need to know about cortisol, is that this hormone does two things: cortisol (together with adrenaline) is the fight-or-flight stress hormone, as well as the body's anti-inflammatory hormone. The concept to embrace here is that both stress and inflammation cause an increase in cortisol; and elevated cortisol in the body is related to almost every major disease.

Most people associate adrenalin as the hormone that we use for stressful situations, and while this is true at the very onset, within fifteen seconds of a stressful event or even a thought, the pituitary gland instructs the adrenal glands to secrete cortisol. A way to understand this is let's say you are absentmindedly walking across a street and you hear the screeching of a car's brakes. Your immediate reaction to avoid getting hit by the car is an adrenalin response. However, if the car is being driven by your ex-spouse and you are now being chased down the street, after fifteen seconds you are literally running on cortisol.

When *The Stress Effect* was initially published there were several research studies linking cortisol to many diseases and health problems, but no-one could explain why such high levels of cortisol were occurring in the general population. Because cortisol was only seen as the stress hormone, the common, knee-jerk explanation for our high cortisol levels focused on how stressed out we had all suddenly become. What was entirely overlooked was the connection between cortisol and its direct relationship to inflammation, and the reasons for the increased inflammation in our bodies.

Over the last decade, a flood of studies have unearthed the missing link: these dramatically rising rates of inflammation in our bodies correlate quite clearly to the increased consumption of fast foods, processed foods, and both over-the-counter and prescription anti-inflammatory pain medication. This is because fast foods and processed foods cause inflammation in our bloodstream, and the anti-inflammatory drugs eventually cause the lining of our intestinal tract to become inflamed. These research studies unequivocally prove the intricate relationship between inflammation, cortisol, health disorders, disease, and—if left untreated—death.

Fast-forward to 2012: hardly a week goes by without a newspaper or magazine telling us about obesity and cortisol, insomnia and cortisol, depression and cortisol, and so on. As a case in point, the May 2012 Reader's Digest informs us of the importance of eating on a regular schedule because, "even eating lunch an hour later than usual can spike levels of the stress hormone cortisol and disrupt your body's ideal state." The February/March 2012 edition of the AARP (American Association of Retired People) tells us that, "chronic stress floods your brain with cortisol, which leads to impaired memory."

The good news since *The Stress Effect*, this book's predecessor, was initially published in 2004 is that there are many exciting and better ways to treat inflammation and cortisol imbalances. The importance given to cortisol imbalances today has risen to the point where there are now doctors who practice what is known as Functional Medicine and Functional Endocrinology, both of which specifically address these imbalances. The bad news is that the list of genetically modified foods, the introduction of high fructose corn syrup, and the changes in our environment that disrupt normal hormone activity all continue to grow and present new health challenges. It's these important changes that prompted me to fully revise and update this book in order to let you know what to watch out for and inform you about the easier approaches now available to correcting these health problems.

One of the main goals of this book is to enable you to look at stress from a totally new perspective. Because stress isn't always a matter of how you respond psychologically and emotionally to the circumstances in your life, but often more to do with the stress hormones coursing through your body on a daily basis in response to internal inflammation. In this book, you'll find clear, easy-to-follow descriptions and flowcharts that show how the vicious cycle of inflammation and cortisol can adversely affect so many functions in your body.

Most books about stress want to convince us that stress and its related symptoms (e.g., insomnia, irritability, upset stomach, diminished libido, etc.) are due to our hectic, multitasking lives, that it's natural to feel emotionally overwhelmed. As a result, we've been led to believe that if we just change our attitudes, meditate, exercise, do yoga for an hour or so every day, we'll no longer be stressed out. Exactly how we're supposed to find the time to fit all of this into our aforementioned hectic, multitasking lives never seems to be a concern in these books.

The idea that stress is completely psychological is scientifically flawed and ignores the role of internal inflammation as a major cause of imbalance in our stress hormone levels. Once again, the hormone that our body secretes in times of stress is the very same hormone it uses to resolve inflammation: cortisol, which is produced by our adrenal glands. The irony here is that taking anti-inflammatory medications—your average, everyday, over-the-counter painkillers—causes intestinal tract inflammation by inhibiting the very enzymes necessary for the intestinal tract to replenish and repair itself, a process that eventually leads to chronic inflammation. The overuse of antibiotics can also cause intestinal tract damage; and the typical, unbalanced American diet of processed foods, fast foods, caffeine, soda, and alcohol further contributes to intestinal tract inflammation, sending inflammatory particles racing around in our bloodstream.

In this book, we're going to look at all the components of stress, and use the holistic model called the *triangle of health* to resolve stress and its harmful effects.

The three components of the triangle are *structural integrity*, *chemical integrity*, and *psychological integrity*. The structural component refers to the health of the body's tissues and the body's alignment; the chemical component refers to diet and hormonal balance; and the psychological component refers to our thoughts and emotional well-being. When all three components are well-balanced, we have optimal health.

Within months of starting my private chiropractic practice thirty-four years ago, it became apparent to me that stress was a major factor in human health disorders. I became fascinated by the way stress affected people so very differently and how there seemed to be some mysterious, hidden factor behind its effects.

I would treat patients who didn't seem to have many actual problems in their lives (besides whatever pain syndrome they were experiencing) but who nonetheless felt totally overwhelmed and stressed out; they were depressed, not sleeping well, craving sugar, salt, and caffeine, and suffering mood swings throughout the day. Then there would be others whose personal lives appeared to be a virtual shipwreck but who—other than suffering the discomfort of backache or neck pain—were doing fine.

Seeing these types of cases over and over again led me to study stress from a perspective open to the notion that perhaps stress wasn't as emotionally-based as it appears on the surface. I began to consider the possibility that maybe much of what I was seeing in these patients who felt so stressed out was due to chemical or structural imbalances that were causing a hypersensitive response to the normal challenges of daily life.

Years of scientific research regarding stress have made it clear that cortisol is a major culprit and the leading chemical factor behind all this suffering. Today, cortisol imbalances have been scientifically linked to obesity, diabetes, depression, heart disease, insomnia, autoimmune diseases like chronic fatigue syndrome, thyroid disorders, ulcers, irritable bowel syndrome, and even osteoporosis.

While it's true that cortisol is the hormone that is secreted when we're either confronted with life-threatening, "fight-or-flight" stress or in a state of emotional distress, might there still be a structural trigger that causes cortisol secretion? As a classic case of which came first, the chicken or the egg, might there not be some structural trigger which initially elevates your cortisol levels, leading you to perceive circumstances in your life as far more stressful than they might seem if your cortisol levels were normal? Well, yes, there is! It's *inflammation*.

Since cortisol is also the body's natural anti-inflammatory chemical, any time there is inflammation, there will be cortisol secretion in response to it. The structural trigger is inflammation, and, again, most of the time it occurs in the intestinal tract as a result of taking anti-inflammatory medications and/or antibiotics, as well as eating a diet that promotes inflammation in the bloodstream.

It's very difficult for most people to relate to this concept of internal inflammation because they think it should cause pain and be obvious, so they discount the idea that they have it. The problem is that we don't have nerve endings to warn us of intestinal tract inflammation or inflammatory chemicals in our bloodstream, so we have no way of knowing. But when you realize that at least 50% of Americans have internal inflammation and the American diet is six times more inflammatory than a normal diet should be, it's not hard to figure out why we're so stressed and sick, and feel like crap.

This book is designed to help you understand all the components of stress and to show you how to correct these imbalances and regain your health. I'm inviting you to take a journey with me and to use my "3R Program" to Resolve inflammation, Repair the intestinal tract, and Restore hormonal balance—and ultimately to see stress in a completely different light. Your experience will be similar to that of a person who doesn't realize how bad her vision is until she puts on a pair of corrective eyeglasses. If your cortisol levels are unbalanced, it can be very difficult to understand that your feelings of being overwhelmed, anxious, depressed, frightened, or worried most of the time are not natural. Your symptoms of fatigue, inability to sleep, food cravings, and weight gain are also not natural, but they can be resolved once you find out what the true cause of these symptoms is.

THE JOURNEY BEGINS

A Chiropractor's Odyssey with Stress

My interest in the adrenal glands, cortisol levels, the human response to stress, inflammation, and the effects of cortisol on health was a gift from my patients. Certainly, endocrine or hormonal systems are studied as part of the anatomy and physiology courses that are taught in chiropractic colleges, but I can't say that at the time, roughly thirty-seven years ago, I found them all that intriguing or particularly relevant to what I thought I would be doing as a practicing chiropractor. Today, the research that I'm presenting regarding inflammation and the cortisol response is widely taught in chiropractic colleges.

While all the aspects of the triangle of health are addressed in chiropractic college, there is no doubt that the emphasis is placed on the structural part, as it's the mission and purpose of chiropractic care to ensure the structural integrity of the body by adjusting or aligning the spinal and peripheral joints. So, with a somewhat limited background in chemical integrity, my real journey deep into the "land of the adrenals" began in my first year of practice with a twenty-eightyear-old male patient suffering multiple joint complaints. It seemed that just about everything hurt: his neck, his lower back, his knees, his elbows, and even his ankles! He was able to function, but the pain was seriously limiting the quality of his life.

After taking a complete history and performing a thorough examination, I initiated a treatment program that consisted of adjusting the painful joints, along with applying cold compresses and performing corrective exercises at home. He responded very well, and the intensity and frequency of his pain progressively diminished to the point where, after one month of care, he was stable and ready to be released from further treatment.

Then one day he came to my office for what I thought would be his last follow-up visit, and nearly all of his symptoms had returned. There was no new injury or accident to account for his pain, and I tried various avenues of questioning in an effort to determine what had caused this sudden recurrence of his symptoms. We went through everything: had he been lifting, gardening, or house cleaning? Had he slept in a poor position? And on and on, with absolutely no clue as to what could be the cause of his recurring pain.

At a loss for any reasonable explanation for a structural cause of his pain, I took a shot at the psychological component and asked if he had encountered any new or unusually stressful situations. It didn't take but a few seconds before he launched into a diatribe about how his little momma from Miami had been visiting for the past two weeks, and she was driving him crazy!

Now, with no disrespect to my own mother, let's just say I had an inkling of (and considerable empathy for), the stress he was experiencing. It gave me my first graphic, clinical insight into how dramatic an effect stress can have on structural alignment and pain. It taught me from then on to always consider a patient's stress profile in determining both the cause and treatment of their problems. With regard to this young man, I gave him a nutritional supplement to support his adrenal glands, and within a few weeks he was fine again.

As the years have passed and stress-related disorders have grown increasingly prevalent, the ways to test for them and use nutritional supplements to address them have become more sophisticated. We now have very accurate saliva tests and blood panels to test for cortisol and other hormone imbalances, food sensitivities, autoimmune diseases, and there are now nutritional supplements that can help lower cortisol levels and balance blood sugar levels.

NO WONDER YOU FEEL LIKE CRAP!

The First Signs of Trouble

When a new patient comes to my office, the first thing I do is sit down with him or her and inquire about the structural, chemical, and, if appropriate, the psychological components of that person's health. Because cortisol can affect nearly every system in our bodies, the list of symptoms associated with cortisol imbalance seems almost endless. The most common ones are cravings for sugar, salt, or carbohydrates; mood swings and irritability; not being able to fall asleep or stay asleep; fluctuation in energy levels throughout the day; allergies and autoimmune diseases; and feeling that the daily demands of life are overwhelming.

One of the most important symptoms of cortisol imbalance I see on a regular basis is insomnia, which is often the first serious indicator of a cortisol imbalance. There are two forms of insomnia: one in which it's hard to fall asleep, and the other in which it's hard to stay asleep.

The problem of initially falling asleep is usually caused by poor blood sugar levels, since our body secretes cortisol to try to balance this out. This patient usually either doesn't eat breakfast or if they do, they are eating cereal, toast, bagels, or pastry, and not getting enough or any protein. The lack of protein as a long burning source of fuel and the overabundance of fast burning carbohydrates means the adrenal glands will secrete cortisol to literally break down muscle tissue (protein) which then get converted into sugar to feed the brain. But this process results in abnormally high levels of cortisol throughout the day and into the evening, and in order to fall asleep cortisol levels should be very low at night. When patients tell me they don't eat protein for breakfast, I sadly break the news to them that they actually **are** eating protein, it's just that they are eating part of themselves.

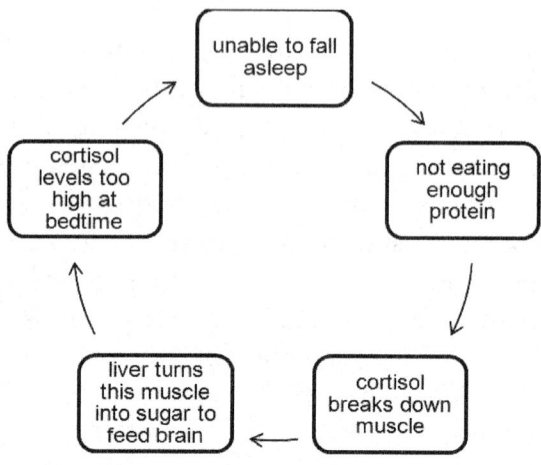

Diagram 1 – First Signs of Trouble – Type 1 Insomnia

In the second type of insomnia, falling asleep is not a problem; but between one and three o'clock in the morning, the patient is wide awake for thirty minutes or longer. This type of insomnia is due to the body's need to repair connective tissue when we're asleep during these hours, and the intestinal tract is considered to be connective tissue. If the intestinal tract is inflamed, then we get the necessary response of cortisol being secreted, and since cortisol is the fight-or-flight hormone, it causes us to become very alert—hence we can't get back to sleep. Probably everyone has experienced this sleep pattern in his or her life when there's a particular worry or stressful situation to deal with, and if it only occurs very occasionally, it's not a big deal. However, in my practice, I see patients who tell me that this is a consistent pattern that they have lived with for years, and for me, as a chiropractor, it has special significance.

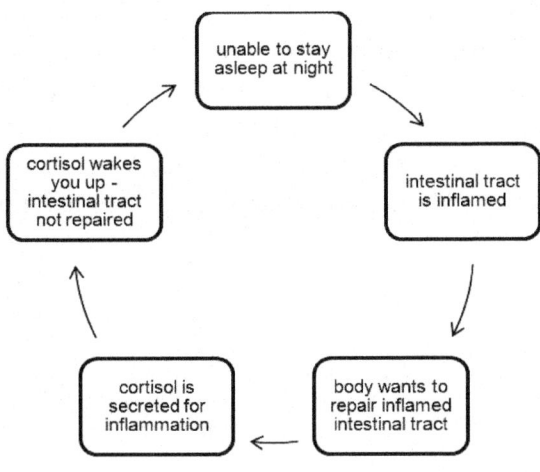

Diagram 2 - Type 2 Insomnia

An obvious part of getting any patient well is the healing process With chiropractic care, the emphasis is on repairing and healing connective tissue—such as ligaments, tendons, and muscles—associated with the joints. It's great to be able to put a misaligned joint back into alignment and restore it to its normal range of motion and mechanical capabilities, but if the connective tissues that hold it in alignment don't properly heal, the joint is likely to pop back out of alignment again.

The connective tissue of the body undergoes a daily repair process while we sleep. Since a consistent pattern of insomnia inhibits the ability of these tissues to heal, the likelihood of achieving joint stability is greatly reduced. And not only is it the connective tissue of joints that are of concern, but once again it's also the intestinal tract lining and other tissues of the body that are not repaired if we're not sleeping.

I never fail to ask a new patient if they have any trouble sleeping, because it often opens up a whole cascade of other hormone-related symptoms and problems, and for me, it's simply not enough to eliminate someone's lower back or neck pain.

Richard Weinstein, D.C.

There are many types of adrenal and related hormone imbalances that I treat on a daily basis, and it's really gratifying to be able to help people get well—not just better, not just symptom-free, but completely well. The success in resolving these cases lies in correlating the components of the triangle of health with the patient's individual symptoms and needs, and in making sure the structural, chemical, and psychological components are well balanced.

THE CORTISOL PARADOX

The Stress and Inflammation Hormone

If we're to make sense of the far-reaching effects of the human stress response and the equally far-reaching effects of inflammation on our bodies, then we're going to have to become acquainted with how this system works. I fully understand that if you're reading this book because you have one of the specific health problems this book covers, perhaps all you really want is to know (metaphorically speaking) what time it is rather than sitting through a lecture on how the clock works. If that's the case, you really could skip ahead to Chapter 6, *Resolving Cortisol Imbalances*, to see how to get started However, for many people, really understanding and grasping the "why" and "how" of their problem is an important step in resolving it, and that's what this chapter is all about.

As with most systems in our bodies, the hormonal system is essentially a feedback loop. This means that we produce specific chemicals to initiate specific reactions, and when they rise to appropriate levels, the system triggers a mechanism to turn it off. This is similar to the relationship between the furnace and thermostat in your home. The thermostat is a temperature-sensitive switch: set to seventy-two degrees, it will signal the furnace to turn on when the ambient temperature drops a tad below this level. As the temperature rises slightly above the desired setting, this again triggers the thermostat, causing it to shut down the furnace. In the human body, this delicate mechanism of balance is referred to as *homeostasis*, and it's largely regulated by the *autonomic nervous system*, which basically controls nearly every bodily function.

Richard Weinstein, D.C.

*The Autonomic Nervous System:
Pedal to the Metal, or Putting on the Brakes*

The underlying neurology that orchestrates the human stress response resides in the autonomic nervous system, which is divided into two branches, one that speeds things up (the *sympathetic*) and one that slows things down (*parasympathetic*). The autonomic nervous system oversees the functions that we don't have to voluntarily control, such as breathing, digestion, blood pressure, blinking, and (for some politicians) thinking. It's important to note, however, that through techniques such as biofeedback and meditation, some of these functions can be consciously controlled.

The sympathetic branch of the autonomic nervous system is the one that gets things going and is activity-oriented. You have sympathetic nerve endings in almost every organ, muscle, and blood vessel to facilitate its function. The adrenal glands also secrete the hormones *epinephrine* and *norepinephrine* to stimulate the sympathetic system in times of stress.

On the other end of the neurological spectrum is the parasympathetic branch, which puts the brakes on the system. It's great to be able to pump out hormones that will increase your heart rate, respiration, blood pressure, and muscle strength for exercise or for responding to physical danger, but you can't go on like that indefinitely without causing trouble. The parasympathetic system is the counterbalance to sympathetic activity that restores calm, promotes relaxation, and facilitates digestive functions, energy storage, and tissue repair and growth. It's the vast difference between these two branches that explains why your parents admonished you as a child not to go swimming until an hour after you had eaten lunch. You run the risk of life-threatening muscle cramping when you try to send your blood to your digestive tract and to skeletal muscles at the same time.

As the sympathetic system becomes engaged in the stress response, be it physiological or psychological, a whole cascade of hormonal events occurs. It's very important to point out that while this system was intended for physical stressors that threatened survival, it operates exactly the same way when the stress is psychological and not life threatening (of course, if you're teaching your teenager to drive, then it's going to be both). The point here is that because the adrenal glands dominate the sympathetic system, you can end up with too much sympathetic activity and too little parasympathetic, causing a host of health problems.

The Limbic System and the Human Response to Stress

The limbic system in the brain is made up of several structures that handle stress, regulate all your hormones, process and store short-term memory, and help in processing emotions and thought. The easiest way to look at the limbic system is as a series of interconnected relay stations that converse with each other in microseconds via a chain reaction of chemicals that cause things to happen. In order to understand stress, we need to look at the limbic system in some detail.

The big players in the limbic system are the *hypothalamus* and the *pituitary gland*, and together they initiate and orchestrate the human response to stress. What happens to them when cortisol levels become unbalanced can dramatically affect your health. You also need to know about them so you will understand what vitamin supplements can be used to support them.

Let's follow an example of a stress response in the life of a typical human being living in a pre-civilized environment like New Jersey. You're walking around, minding your own business, looking for a few grubs or berries to eat, and you hear a sound like the snapping of a branch or the rustling of leaves.

Your body's first response is to have your limbic system evaluate the information it has just received. Maybe it's just the wind, or maybe it's a predator that thinks you might make a good lunch—and we're not talking about your culinary skills here. Your limbic system processes this information to determine the significance of this stimulus. If it decides that danger is present, then you're hormonally off to the races, and I mean that literally. The hypothalamus kicks into action and secretes a messenger-like substance that then causes the pituitary gland to secrete another messenger-like substance, which in turn causes the adrenal glands to secrete cortisol.

Cortisol is such an elegantly effective hormone that, like a courier of old bearing the King's seal, it can affect virtually every system in the body—an excellent way of orchestrating the body's expenditure of energy when survival is threatened. But as we will discover, the very thing that makes cortisol so powerful also makes it devastatingly dangerous when levels remain either too high or too low for prolonged periods of time.

Now back to lunch, where you're about to become the main course. You have now entered the fight or flight decision tree, and either you're going to have a physical confrontation or you're going to try to outrun the predator and become a genetic ancestor of a future Boston marathon winner. The first thing you're going to need to accomplish either of these tasks is fuel, which in this case means *glucose* (or, plainly put, sugar).

The release of cortisol will immediately stimulate a process known as *glucogenesis* (*gluco*= sugar + *genesis*= making of something, thus literally the making of sugar; this process becomes critical when we get into blood sugar problems, cholesterol, diet, weight gain, and insomnia). During glucogenesis, the body makes glucose from protein amino acids in the liver. In a stress response, cortisol can increase the rate of glucose production by **six to ten** times the normal rate, dramatically increasing the availability of the fuel your muscles are going to need to get out of this dangerous predicament.

So now we have the fuel delivery system, but we still need oxygen to make it work. It's time for cortisol to affect your cardiovascular system by narrowing your arteries while at the same time the epinephrine from the adrenal glands increases your heart rate. By pumping blood harder and faster through a narrower channel, you have increased your blood pressure and increased the flow of oxygen-enriched blood to your muscles. You have now mobilized the glucose and oxygen you need for the impending 100-yard dash or a few rounds fighting a grizzly bear.

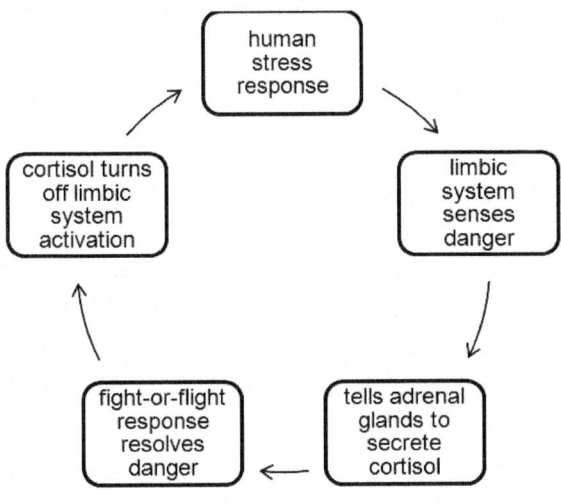

Diagram 3 - the Autonomic Nervous System

Once the stress is resolved, the cortisol circulates back to the hypothalamus, and the emergency system shuts down. With chronic or repetitive stress, however, the hypothalamus gets bombarded with too much cortisol; it can then can lose its sensitivity to cortisol and be unable to stop the pituitary gland from signaling the adrenal glands to keep secreting cortisol. This means the shut-off switch for cortisol is broken and chronically elevated levels of cortisol occur. This is like the thermostat in your home malfunctioning so that it no longer knows when it's hot enough and isn't able to turn off the furnace.

The Adrenal Gland Hormones

It's now time to get acquainted with the cortisol factory in the human stress response, your adrenal glands. You have two of them, and they sit on top of each of your kidneys. The adrenal glands have two distinct parts: the *innermost medulla*, which comprises twenty percent of the gland, and the *outer cortex*.

The adrenal medulla is related to the sympathetic nervous system, and its job is to secrete the hormones epinephrine and norepinephrine. These hormones keep the bronchiole tubes in the lungs clear and promote the ability to concentrate, so you can see what a lack of these hormones can cause: asthma and poor concentration (ADD, or Attention Deficit Disorder and ADHD, or Attention Deficit Hyperactivity Disorder).

The cortex produces three types of hormones: one that regulates the minerals in your body such as sodium, potassium, and magnesium; cortisol, which we now know manages stress and inflammation but also is very important in regulating sugar, protein, and fat metabolism; and sex hormones such as DHEA.

The sex hormones produced by the cortex play different roles, but the most important one is *dehydroepiandrosterone*, which fortunately for all of us has been abbreviated to DHEA. Much has been written about DHEA over the past several years, touting it as everything from the fountain of youth to the cure for cancer. The problem with most of these claims is that they fail to look at the bigger picture and how DHEA functions in a relative balance with cortisol. Taking oral doses of DHEA (available in any vitamin store) in the hope it will make you younger, sexier, or stronger, without first addressing any imbalance in cortisol levels, is at best futile and at worst dangerous.

The reason DHEA received such notoriety as the "youth" hormone is because the adrenal glands produce the greatest quantities of it between the ages of seven and twenty-five. As we age, there is a progressive decline in DHEA production, and by age seventy-five, we're only producing fifteen to twenty percent of what we were back in our peak years. So it's seductive to think that all you have to do is increase your levels of DHEA, and you'll return to being the horny and crazy adolescent you once were. While this may be a great way to sell pills, it doesn't take into account the many factors that can cause DHEA production to be too low.

A very important feature of DHEA and cortisol secretion is that under normal circumstances they follow a predictable *circadian rhythm*, or twenty-four-hour cycle. Cortisol levels should be high in the early morning, peak around eight A.M., and then progressively decline until they reach their lowest level in the evening. In order to maintain balance, DHEA production follows a daily, circadian cycle which is the opposite to that of cortisol.

Another hormone, *melatonin*, has a twenty-four hour rhythm that is also exactly the opposite of cortisol, and melatonin helps us sleep. As cortisol levels should be declining throughout the day, the DHEA and melatonin levels should be rising. This is important, because if your adrenal glands are producing elevated amounts of cortisol late at night, you'll develop insomnia; you will, as mentioned earlier, either have trouble falling asleep, or else fall asleep just fine but find yourself waking up two and a half to three hours later and then have difficulty getting back to sleep. Sometimes you'll lie awake staring at the ceiling for a half hour; other times it will take several hours before you finally return to sleep.

This disruptive sleep pattern creates a twofold problem. The first includes the physiological and psychological consequences of sleep deprivation, i.e., fatigue and depression. The second is that your body conducts most of its repair functions during sleep, and the inability to consistently restore worn or damaged cells will result in pain and illness.

Why Elevated Cortisol Levels can be Dangerous

While the secretion of cortisol orchestrates the response to stress and flips all of the right switches for fight or flight, the effects of cortisol aren't quite done with you yet. Since your body knows that at this critical moment your only agenda is survival, it decides to shut down other functions that might divert energy from your fight-or-flight response.

One of the principal effects of cortisol on the metabolism is the reduction of protein stores in essentially all body cells except those of the liver. During the stress response the proteins in the liver are being turned into glucose for fuel, but everywhere else in the body protein is either being broken down, or its production has stopped. Your body figures there is no point in storing or making new protein if you're going to be dead in two minutes, so it takes a wait-and-see approach.

Why is this dangerous? Because **during a stress response your body will not engage in tissue growth or repair.** As you can imagine, this can have dramatic consequences if you have chronically high levels of cortisol in response to inflammation rather than actual stress. You will find it hard to repair tissues or recover from injuries, and will injure yourself more easily.

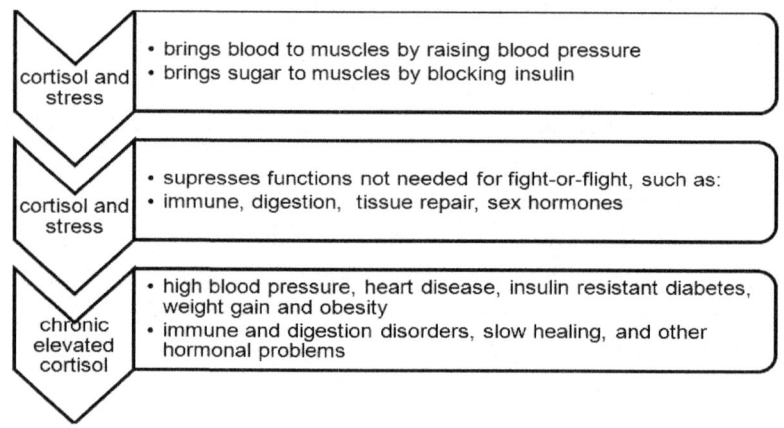

Diagram 4 - Cortisol and Stress Response

Cortisol and Sex

Another effect of elevated cortisol is the depletion of the reproductive system. Let's say you're a twenty-eight-year-old male being chased by a predator, and you happen to run by a stream where young women are bathing. Clearly, this is not the appropriate time to achieve an erection. Your body is far more concerned about whether you will still be alive in the next five minutes than whether you might be engaging in sexual activity anytime in the near future, so it (wisely) sees no point in making the reproductive hormones. If the stress goes on for too long, a common problem among males is impotence.

As for females, increased stress can both inhibit the libido and put the brakes on ovulation. This can happen in several ways. As Jay Kaplan of Bowman Grey Medical School has demonstrated, stress can suppress the estrogen levels of female monkeys as effectively as removing their ovaries. It also appears that while the adrenal glands are busy producing cortisol and epinephrine for stress, they are diverted from making the *androgenic* (male) sex hormones (it's known that the sex drive can be diminished by surgically removing the adrenal glands, and can be restored with the administration of synthetic androgens).

Cortisol and the Immune System

In the same way that your body disarms its repair and reproductive systems during stress, the immune system is also inhibited as part of the stress response. This occurs in several different ways, but mostly it's cortisol that is responsible for suppressing the immune system's ability to function.

On a very basic level, the immune system is comprised of white blood cells which are responsible for roaming around the body looking for infectious invading cells and foreign objects to attack and kill. For the purpose of simplicity, we'll focus on the immune cells that come from the *thymus gland* and are therefore called *T-cells*. There are also chemical messengers called *interleukins* which help the T-cells differentiate between invading microbes that need to be attacked and the body's own tissue.

There are many ways in which stress and, in particular, cortisol, inhibit the immune system:

- Cortisol can keep white blood cells in the thymus gland from becoming T-cells, and can even cause the thymus gland to shrink.

- Cortisol suppresses the release of the interleukin messengers, which makes the T-cells either less responsive or, worse, causes them to make mistakes and attack your own tissue, triggering what is called an autoimmune disease.

- Last, but certainly not least, cortisol can just flat-out **kill** the white blood cells by entering them and destroying their DNA.

Considering all of the ways stress can dismember the immune system, it's not hard to understand why people get sick after a period of stress. Nearly everyone can relate to the experience of getting sick after taking final exams or on their honeymoon or on vacation from a stressful job.

Cortisol: the Body's Anti-Inflammatory Agent

By now you probably think cortisol is the demon hormone that made that little girl's head spin around in The Exorcist, but it's not that simple. One of the positive effects of cortisol, other than potentially saving your behind in a fight-or-flight situation, is that it's a powerful anti-inflammatory agent. Understanding the relationship of cortisol to inflammation is critically important, and is very often a big piece of the puzzle when things really go awry in the body.

Inflammation of the body's tissue can be caused by a number of things, including:

- Trauma

- Infections

- Prolonged use of substances such as *nonsteroidal anti-inflammatory drugs* (NSAIDS), antibiotic drugs, alcohol, caffeine, phosphoric acid (some sodas)

- A diet high in *omega-6 oils* (found in processed foods, fast foods, and junk foods), which cause elevated levels of inflammatory chemicals

All these factors will cause internal inflammation; in some cases, such as rheumatoid arthritis, the inflammation is the most damaging part of the disease. As an example that's easy to relate to, let's take your nose. Your darling child comes home from preschool as a carrier of every germ known to the National Institutes of Health and gives you a big hug and a kiss. These germs now enter your system either orally or as airborne messengers of disease. If your immune system is not up to the challenge, these microbes will set up camp in your throat or nasal passage and begin to multiply. At some point, specialized cells in your immune system, called *mast cells*, will become aware of the invading organisms, yell, "Mayday! Mayday!" and then explode. The purpose of this is to release *histamine*, which will cause inflammation in order to attract the white blood cells of your immune system and so launch the holy war in your mucous membranes. At this point, tissues in hand, you head for the drugstore in search of antihistamine nasal sprays or pills to reduce the inflammation and swelling.

As we've already discussed, cortisol can suppress the immune system. At first you might think this is a stupid action on your body's part, and no wonder your cold seems to last for weeks. Here you're taking echinacea, goldenseal, and God knows what else to build up your immune system, and those knuckleheaded adrenal glands are producing cortisol to suppress it! Well, this is where homeostasis (balance) comes in.

Cortisol affects inflammation in several ways. It stabilizes the membranes of the cells that release the *proteolytic enzymes*, histamines, and *prostaglandins* that cause inflammation; and by reducing the permeability of the small blood vessels, cortisol also restricts the transport of these inflammatory chemicals throughout the body. An example of cortisol's powerful effect on inflammation, especially if you have ever had poison ivy or poison oak rashes, is the prescription drug called *cortisone*, which is pharmaceutical synthetic cortisol.

An unchecked immune system responding to unabated inflammation will probably eat you up over time and turn into an autoimmune disease, as a result of which your immune system begins attacking normal cells. So in appropriate amounts, cortisol carries out damage control by reducing the inflammation and also by not allowing the immune system to get overly aggressive. In a similar vein (no pun intended), the reduction in permeability of the small blood vessels reduces the migration of the white blood cells throughout the body, which again regulates the immune response.

Another aspect of cortisol's participation in the immune response is that it can lower fever by inhibiting the release of *interleukin-1*, which besides being an immune system messenger is also the chemical that excites the body's temperature control. Having a fever when you're sick is a great defense mechanism, because it's your body's way of trying to create an environment that the invading microbes can't live in. But in the wisdom of homeostasis and in an effort to not cook your brain cells, cortisol can keep this process from getting out of control.

There's no doubt that proper levels of cortisol are crucial to orchestrating the appropriate response to life-threatening stress or to managing inflammation and the immune system. But what happens if the stress (physical, psychological, or a combination of both) becomes chronic, or the inflammation becomes chronic, or the stress and the inflammation get caught up in a vicious dance with each other?

PHYSICAL STRESS AND THE PRO-INFLAMMATORY DIET

There's a Fire Down Below

Let's go step-by-step down the road of how your body became inflamed in the first place and see what happens to it and to your health as the inflammation progresses.

Because the inflammation in question is invisible, it's frightening how many people end up feeling like crap without a clue as to how they got there. I see this all the time in my practice.

For most of my patients who have cortisol imbalances there is usually a history of taking over-the-counter pain medications (NSAIDS such as aspirin or ibuprofen) for quite a while; of repeated use of antibiotics for infections (often since early childhood with multiple ear infections); of a diet with way too much soda and junk food; and often of combinations of the above. In the end, this lifestyle produces a real physical stress on the body and results in an inescapable vicious cycle.

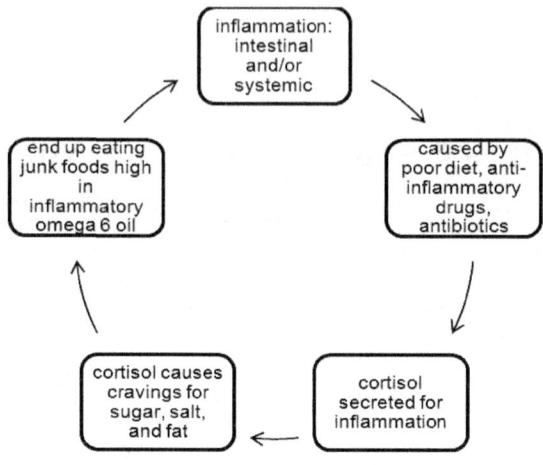

Diagram 5 - Inflammation and Cortisol

In its classic interpretation, physical stress is usually correlated with the fight-or-flight survival response. However, other physical stressors, such as pain and (more importantly) inflammation, cause cortisol levels to rise to the point at which they can become chronic and dangerous. Inflammation and the damage it causes to the body have been ignored for far too long by the medical community. Recent research, however, has shown how serious inflammation can be, and new federal recommendations are being written that urge doctors to test for it.

In fact, inflammation is now attracting a great deal of attention from medical researchers who consider it to be an even bigger factor in heart disease than cholesterol. In a research paper published in the New England Journal of Medicine, Dr. Paul Ridker of Boston's Brigham and Women's Hospital states that up to thirty-five million Americans have normal cholesterol but above average levels of inflammation, putting them at unusual risk for heart attacks and strokes. The reason for the risk of heart disease isn't the inflammation by itself, but the cortisol response to inflammation and the fact that cortisol raises blood pressure.

Causes of Inflammation

Interestingly enough, Dr. Paul Ridker's paper never determines where all this inflammation is coming from, but chronic intestinal tract inflammation is known to be caused by the overuse of nonsteroidal anti-inflammatory drugs (NSAIDs), caffeinated beverages, alcohol, antibiotics, mental stress, or any combination of these factors.

The other cause of inflammation is going to be the *pro-inflammatory diet*, in which the consumption of foods high in omega-6 oils causes elevated levels of highly inflammatory chemicals. Sadly, this describes the typical American diet of fast foods, junk foods, fried foods, and processed foods. While intestinal tract inflammation is specific to one organ, the pro-inflammatory diet results in *systemic inflammation*, the result of a highly inflammatory chemical circulating through the bloodstream. In my opinion, the medical researchers involved with inflammation find themselves in a quandary regarding the revelation of the causes of inflammation, as they are probably not thrilled about taking on either the pharmaceutical or fast food industries.

Remember, the human response to stress is designed to handle short-term stress, since all of the biochemical processes are clearly meant for managing a fight-or-flight response. After all, just how long do you think it takes to either run from or fight a tiger? It obviously wouldn't benefit the survival of a species to develop a mechanism for stress management that can shut down its own repair and growth processes, reproductive functions, and immune system, if it wasn't designed around the idea that the stress would be relatively short-term.

The Beginning of Trouble

So how does the physical stress of inflammation or injury cause elevated levels of stress hormones? I want to take you through a few scenarios that occur with alarming regularity and which illustrate how cortisol imbalances get started, how they can spiral out of control, and how devastating is their effect on human health. I want to show you *why* you feel like crap.

You lift something improperly, spend too much time in the garden bent over pulling weeds, slip and fall down, get into a car accident, or injure yourself in a sporting activity, and now you're in pain. The pain isn't going away as quickly as you'd hoped it would, and as a good, television-abiding American you want "fast, fast, fast relief." You go to your medicine cabinet and choose from any number of NSAIDs that are lined up on the shelves. There are an amazing number of NSAIDs available, of which the most popular are:

- Ibuprofen (e.g., Motrin, Advil)
- Aspirin (e.g., Bayer, Anacin, Bufferin)
- Naproxen (e.g., Aleve, Anaprox)
- Piroxicam (e.g., Feldene)
- Sulindac (e.g., Clinoril)
- Diclofenac (e.g., Voltaren)

An exception to this list is acetaminophen (Tylenol), which is an analgesic pain reliever which doesn't affect inflammation.

NSAIDs relieve inflammation in much the same way cortisol does: by blocking the release of prostaglandins and *arachidonic acid*. So far, so good.

But what if your injury doesn't improve, and you continue to take them for an extended period of time?

- There are several research studies that have looked into this question, and their conclusions are staggering. Swiss researchers report that NSAIDs are killing **at leas**t 2,000 patients each year in the United Kingdom because of bleeding ulcers. The researchers say that NSAIDs block the production of a *coenzyme* called *cox-1* that protects the mucous lining of the stomach. This study suggests that about 1 in 1,000 patients who take these drugs as prescribed regularly for two years **will die** from them.

- A study published by Stanford University School of Medicine in April 1999 paints an even darker picture. This study states: "Nonsteriodal anti-inflammatory drugs are one of the most commonly used classes of medications worldwide. It's estimated that more than 30 million people in the US take NSAIDs daily. Gastrointestinal inflammation related to NSAID therapy is the most prevalent category of adverse drug reactions."

- The statistics that the Stanford study reveals are truly alarming:

- In this country, 103,000 people are hospitalized yearly due to intestinal tract inflammation caused by NSAIDs, at an average cost of $15,000 to $20,000 per case.

- An average of **16,500 deaths** occur in the United States every year from intestinal-tract inflammation and bleeding caused by NSAIDs (compared to this country's yearly rate of 16,685 deaths caused by HIV, or Human Immunodeficiency Virus.

- If NSAID-related deaths were tabulated separately in the National Vital Statistics report, it would be the fifteenth most common cause of death in the United States, putting it far ahead of deaths caused by Hodgkin's disease, ovarian cancer, and asthma.

- Only one out of five people who have serious intestinal-tract inflammation will have any warning signs.

Now here comes the really scary part: the statistics from this Stanford study account only for people who have been **prescribed** NSAIDs by their medical doctors for arthritis. The study did not take into account all of the people who regularly take over-the-counter NSAIDs for headaches, back pain, or other pain syndromes.

By examining the effects of NSAIDs on the digestive tract we can see the origin of the adrenal dilemma:

- You're in pain, which means there's likely to be some degree of inflammation involved, and you're taking NSAIDs.

- However, because the NSAIDs are only treating the symptoms and not the cause of your pain, the pain persists, and you continue to take the NSAIDs to relieve your symptoms.

- The NSAIDs are now inhibiting the prostaglandin production you need to repair your digestive tract on a daily basis from the onslaught of acids and enzymes necessary to digest your food.

- As the protective mucous lining of your digestive tract becomes degraded, the walls of the digestive tract become inflamed, so now you have even more inflammation in your body than you started with.

Can you guess what your adrenal glands are up to by now? You'll recall that the adrenal glands will produce cortisol in any stress response, including tissue injury and inflammation. But cortisol, like NSAIDs, also inhibits the production of the prostaglandins that repair the digestive tract, so at this point the inflammation in your digestive tract is going to get progressively worse, causing even higher levels of cortisol to be produced, which will simply exacerbate the problem. You have begun the odyssey into the nightmare land of *chronic adrenal stress*, a vicious cycle of pain, increased cortisol levels, the inability to repair tissue damage and inflammation, and more pain.

Leaky Gut Syndrome

After your gastrointestinal tract has been inflamed for several months and the tissue lining has become progressively eroded, the next step in this process is the occurrence of microscopic holes in the intestinal wall, which will cause the wall to become abnormally porous and to leak incompletely digested bits of food, microbes, and toxins into your system. Commonly referred to as *leaky gut syndrome*, a condition in which metabolic and microbial toxins escape from the small intestines and flood into the bloodstream, this condition has at least two negative consequences.

The first consequence of leaky gut syndrome is that the incompletely digested particles of food and microbes escaping from the small intestinal lining will trigger an immune system response. Any time a foreign object enters the body, it's the responsibility of the immune system and its trusty T-cells to attack it, and most of the time this process works efficiently.

With leaky gut syndrome, the immune system perceives these escaping food particles as dangerous viruses and mounts an attack. At the same time, viruses and bacteria are also leaking out of the intestines, and the immune system is going to have to deal with them as well. This puts a continuous strain on the immune system, and the immune system response becomes an exercise in futility because, as long as the intestinal tract is leaking and you keep eating, your immune system is never going to be able to get ahead of the toxins.

To help complicate matters further, the adrenal glands are still producing elevated levels of cortisol in response to the intestinal tract inflammation and, as we discussed in the previous chapter, cortisol works to suppress the immune system. If this goes on for a prolonged period of time, the immune system will begin to break down.

The second negative consequence of leaky gut syndrome concerns the liver's ability to detoxify your body. Think of your liver as a waste-management treatment plant that is responsible for screening out all the junk circulating in your body. The process by which your liver does this is called *stage two detoxification*, and it works as follows:

- All the blood circulating in the body must pass through the liver before it returns to the lungs and heart. As the blood passes through, the liver removes toxic waste material.

- If the toxins are water soluble, the kidneys are responsible for excreting them in the urine.

- If they are fat soluble, the liver sends the toxins through the common bile duct of the gallbladder, which is located directly under the liver, and the bile duct carries the toxins to the small intestinal tract.

- The toxins that end up in the intestinal tract will then be processed by a combination of digestive enzymes and healthy microbes before being eliminated in a bowel movement.

But remember, in our current scenario the wall of the intestinal tract has microscopic holes in it and cannot contain the toxins being transported to it by the liver, resulting in a toxic merry-go-round. The very toxins that the liver is trying to remove keep circulating back to it over and over again, thereby creating continuous stress on the liver and gallbladder duct. A further problem is that the liver is also responsible for the activation of some hormones, such as *thyroid* and *estrogen*, and if it's worn out and depleted of enzymes, it can't do it and you can develop disorders such as *hypothyroidism* (decreased thyroid function) or menstrual problems.

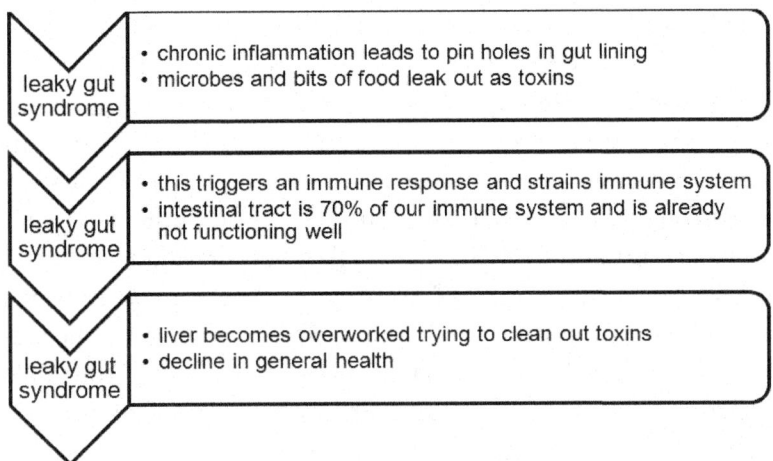

Diagram 6 - Leaky Gut Syndrome

Unfortunately, you're probably still experiencing the pain that got you started taking the NSAIDs in the first place, since they only mask the symptoms and don't correct the cause of back pain, neck pain, or headaches. As you may recall from Chapter 2, the normal secretion of cortisol follows a daily circadian rhythm in which the cortisol level is highest in the morning and lowest at night. Elevated levels of cortisol at night result in insomnia. So now your body can't repair itself very well because the elevated levels of cortisol are suppressing your body's natural repair mechanisms and disrupting your normal sleep, which is the time your body should be carrying out the repair process.

So your digestive tract is inflamed from all the NSAIDs you're taking and leaking all manner of toxins into your bloodstream, and your immune system is being suppressed and overworked at the same time. You aren't sleeping at night and you're probably craving sugar, salt, or both due to the excess cortisol inhibiting your insulin and weakening the adrenal glands' ability to make the hormone that regulates your body's mineral content. Your life is not exactly wonderful.

You have plenty of physical problems, which by now are probably causing some mental stress. You don't feel well, and you're beginning to worry that maybe you're never going to feel well ever again. You're not sleeping well because the elevated cortisol level causes you to wake up around two o'clock in the morning, and you toss and turn for an hour or more before you can get back to sleep—so now you're tired and cranky to boot. Your blood sugar is bouncing up and down, which makes you crave and eat foods that end up making you feel even worse. You're gaining weight as a result of eating the carbohydrates you're craving and because you can't exercise due to the pain you're experiencing. You're also experiencing mood swings, and are either easily agitated and argumentative, or withdrawn and depressed, or both at varying times.

By now you really do feel like crap; sadly, it can still get worse.

Given the fact that you're run down and your immune system is overtaxed, the next misfortune you're likely to encounter is that you begin getting sick more often with colds, influenza, or other infections. This will bring you to your medical doctor and a probable course of antibiotic therapy.

The problem with antibiotics is that they destroy the beneficial bacteria living in your small and large intestines. The intestinal tract has over five hundred different kinds of beneficial bacteria that perform hundreds of functions necessary for a healthy metabolism and immune response. Through enzyme secretions, bacteria transform metabolic and microbial wastes before these are discharged in a bowel movement. If you already have an inflamed intestinal tract and subsequent leaky gut syndrome from too many NSAIDs, taking antibiotics will only further impair your ability to purge toxins from your system.

If all this is happening to you and you happen to be a woman, you're likely to experience even further complications in your hormonal balance because the amount of estrogen that gets released into your system is regulated by the liver and the bacteria in the intestinal tract. The liver sends excess estrogen through the gallbladder duct to the small intestines, where the normal bacteria break it down. If you lack the bacteria to destroy excess estrogen and you have intestinal leakage, the estrogen will be reabsorbed and can end up in estrogen receptor sites such as the breasts, ovaries, and uterus. This may contribute to fibroid tumors, estrogen sensitive cancers, premenstrual syndrome (PMS), and monthly migraines related to menstrual cycles.

Candida Yeast Infections

Should you continue on either a prolonged or repetitive course of antibiotic therapy, you'll graduate to another problem, which is a *Candida* infection in the intestinal tract. *Candida Albicans* is a yeast that, under normal circumstances, inhabits the intestinal tract in relative balance with the rest of the intestinal microbes. Unfortunately, the antibiotics will kill the normal bacteria that serve to keep the Candida population in check. The Candida cells excrete a chemical that shrinks the cells of the intestinal wall, and as these cells continue to wither away, the intestinal tract further degrades, becomes more inflamed, and leaks even more toxins into the bloodstream.

So now you have a Candida infection, and the yeast is living off the carbohydrates you're eating, which results in a further imbalance in your blood sugar levels. Remember that an elevated level of cortisol will inhibit your cells' sensitivity to insulin and your ability to store glucose for energy; now the Candida is living off your glucose-producing foods before you can even use them, and your energy level is dropping because your muscles and brain are starved for the glucose that fuels them. Your sugar cravings are increasing; you're consuming lots of junk food that is high in calories; and you're probably gaining more weight.

You obviously are still not getting well. You still have pain; you seem to get sick every other week; and your friends, loved ones, and the people you work with are starting to think you're a hypochondriac. You're missing work because of your multiple illnesses, and when you're there, you're not very productive. But at least things can't get any worse. Or can they?

Richard Weinstein, D.C.

Autoimmune Attacks

This is a good time to recall that cortisol suppresses the part of the immune system that is responsible for preventing an autoimmune attack. Your immune system knows which cells belong to you and which ones don't (and therefore are worthy of killing) by a process called *self-tolerance*. Self-tolerance is regulated by cells produced in the thymus gland and bone marrow, with the interleukins mentioned above acting as messengers to the killer T-cells. Prolonged periods of elevated cortisol levels can destroy immune system cells, rob these cells of the chemicals that are necessary for them to function properly, and even shrink the thymus gland that is making these immune system cells. Add this to the fact that your poor immune system is already overburdened by dealing with the toxins leaking out of your intestinal tract, and this might provide an excellent opportunity to develop an autoimmune disease.

Very recent research now tells us that you cannot have an autoimmune disease without having leaky gut syndrome first. The overworked, poorly-formed immune cells begin to make mistakes and start attacking the body's own tissues, resulting in diseases such as rheumatoid arthritis, fibromyalgia, thyroid disease, and multiple sclerosis. I will discuss autoimmune diseases in greater detail a little later when we delve into cortisol's role in specific diseases.

When Katrina came to see me as a patient she had one of the worst and most complicated cases of rheumatoid arthritis I had ever seen. It began two and a half years previously with extreme fatigue and an all-over ache in her joints; she said it felt as though she had the flu all the time. Then the joints in her feet began to swell and become disfigured and she developed a lump growing out of her lower forearm. Her digestive tract hurt, and she would bloat after eating. Her medical doctors performed blood tests and arrived at a diagnosis of rheumatoid arthritis, but all the drug therapies failed miserably. She was given several medications for rheumatoid arthritis and—in a last-ditch effort—she was even given intravenous drugs. Yet nothing worked and she became progressively worse. After two and a half years her doctors told her there was nothing else they could think of other than to put her on anti-depressant medication. By the time she came to see me, she looked at least fifteen years older than her age of forty-nine.

The first area of interest for me was her intestinal tract, and for her illness to be so bad I immediately came up with the idea that not only must she have a severely leaky gut, but by now she would also test positive for food sensitivities. Food sensitivities are different from a food allergy in that an allergy will probably bring about a immune reaction like a skin rash; food sensitivities don't cause a rash but instead cause the immune cells in the intestinal tract (remember, your intestinal tract is **70%** of your whole immune system) to flare up and attack particles of food. It turns out that the food particles most likely to trigger an immune attack are the ones you eat most often. This process is inflammatory, and you know what that means—more cortisol.

As it turned out, Katrina had food sensitivities to nearly 90% of all of the foods she was regularly eating. But it wasn't only foods, she also had sensitivities to most of her cosmetics and even her toothpaste, which explained why her gums would bleed every time she brushed her teeth, even though her dentist ruled out periodontal disease. So the first thing I had to do with her was clear out the food and chemical sensitivities, since I knew that her intestinal tract would never repair itself with all the immune cell "wars" going on in there.

(This often isn't as hard as it sounds because the average person usually has a fairly rigid diet, even without knowing they do. To check this for yourself, write down everything you eat for two weeks and see if the same foods don't keep popping up on your list. Remember to look for what is called cross-referencing, which means nothing more than the fact that potatoes are still potatoes no matter how many different ways you prepare them, and wheat is still wheat whether it's pasta, pizza, sandwiches, pancakes, bagels, or ravioli. The best way to scientifically test for cross-referencing sensitivities is through the Cryex Lab test for it—see the Resource Guide at the end of the book).

So I had Katrina make up the same list I just asked you to, and, sure enough, as a very busy working mother, a lot of the same foods came up week after week. Sometimes having children who are picky eaters contributes to this problem, because if you can only get them to eat two proteins, three vegetables, and two grains, it's always the same basic menu week after week. Clearing the sensitivities means getting the patient to stop eating what they usually eat and start eating things they ideally never, or almost never eat, because the immune cells in the intestinal tract literally do not recognize these food particles and will not attack them.

While she was changing her entire approach to food, I had her stop or change the cosmetics she was using and stop using toothpaste for a while and switch to baking soda. Then I started her on my 3R Program—<u>R</u>epair the intestinal tract; <u>R</u>esolve inflammation; <u>R</u>estore hormonal balance (all this is discussed in great detail in Chapter 6).

While I was certainly hoping Katrina's case would improve, I couldn't have imagined that in five weeks her joint pain and fatigue would be gone, her stomach would feel fine, and her gums would stop bleeding. She looked like a completely different woman and, as she still had her regular appointments with her other three doctors, found that they could not get over how great she looked. By eight weeks her blood tests for rheumatoid arthritis were normal.

Adrenal Fatigue

Tom was a sixty-year-old office worker under continuous work stress for years, which resulted in poor eating and sleeping habits. He was certainly looking forward to retirement, but it occurred earlier than planned when he contracted mononucleosis (mono as it's commonly referred to) and became so ill that he had to quit working. By the time he came to see me two years later, he had seen several other doctors and the last diagnosis he came away with was adrenal fatigue. Although he had done a good job of eliminating sugar and all wheat (gluten) from his diet, he was constantly tired and always needed to nap during the day; he couldn't stay asleep at night, and he just had no energy or enthusiasm for life. He was taking sixteen different vitamin supplements recommended by the host of other doctors he had seen that were supposed to correct his condition, and none of them helped. He came to see me after he read this book (the original 2004 edition).

NO WONDER YOU FEEL LIKE CRAP!

The first thing that went wrong in Tom's attempt to get well was that no-one bothered to check the status of his intestinal tract. So I had him do the ASI *test (Adrenal Stress Index test, fully discussed in the next chapter). The results showed that besides his cortisol levels being very low throughout the entire day, his intestinal tract was seriously inflamed. The final straw that led him to his present condition was that the intestinal tract's constant state of inflammation put such a demand on his adrenal glands that it eventually wore them out. He still had enough adrenal function to have the middle-of-the-night cortisol response to the intestinal tract inflammation wake him up, but that was about all his adrenals could manage.*

So Tom's treatment protocol with me started with the critically important first R, Repair the intestinal tract. As long as his intestinal tract was inflamed, he was never going to be able to digest and **absorb** *all of the good organic food he had changed his diet to, not to mention the sixteen vitamin supplements he was told to take. After just four weeks his intestinal tract healed, he was sleeping fine, and I added the rest of the 3R Program knowing he would be able to absorb the supplements I wanted him to take. He phoned me three weeks later to tell me that he was feeling great, had lots of energy and no longer needed any naps, and decided he wanted to donate his time to a children's charity.*

This brings us to the other side of the problem with adrenal gland disorders, which is that it's not always a matter of producing too much cortisol, but also too little. This is known as *adrenal fatigue*, and it's the last phase of *adrenal dysfunction*. This occurs in some people when there has been a chronic demand for cortisol for so long that at some point the adrenal glands can no longer make enough cortisol for even normal function.

A deficiency in cortisol will make it impossible to maintain normal blood sugar levels throughout the day. As discussed earlier, cortisol is necessary for the process known as glucogenesis—the conversion of proteins into usable glucose—and an abnormal reduction of cortisol results in lowered blood sugar levels. This is a clear example of why it's so important for the cortisol levels to be normal: because if they are too high, cortisol inhibits insulin utilization so that you can't metabolize the carbohydrates you eat into usable glucose; and if they are too low, you can't convert proteins into glucose. Either way your blood sugar is too low, which all by itself can cause fatigue, headaches, irritability, and sugar cravings.

Another effect of insufficient cortisol is the inability to access proteins and fats from the body's tissues, which depresses many other metabolic functions. This creates a sluggish metabolism even if plenty of glucose and nutrients are otherwise available to the muscles. The lack of cortisol will make the muscles weak and dysfunctional.

Inadequate cortisol secretion also makes the body more susceptible to the harmful effects of stress, increasing the likelihood of infections and difficulty in getting over them. Once again, this is an excellent example of the need for homeostasis or balance; too much or too little cortisol has a negative effect on the immune system. This is one of those chicken or egg situations: are you stressed out because you're sick, or are you sick because you're stressed?

While people with cortisol levels that are too high have a hair-trigger response to stress and fly off the handle with the least bit of provocation, people whose cortisol levels are too low are also unable to deal with stress appropriately and are easily overwhelmed. They are literally sick and tired, and the simple tasks of everyday life become magnified into problems they can't deal with. Their sodium and glucose levels are unstable, causing them to crave salt and/or sugar; their muscles are getting progressively weaker; their immune system is sliding further downhill; and their ability to have a normal and productive life is seriously compromised.

This is the point at which chronic fatigue syndrome is likely to occur.

Diet, Inflammation, and Hormone Imbalance

The inability to recover from an injury or to resolve a pain syndrome, the repetitive use of NSAIDs, and the overuse of antibiotics are not the only ways to end up with unbalanced cortisol levels. Another scenario is that of a chronically poor diet. **Poor diet can be a major player in causing hormonal imbalances**, and it can do so on several levels. So here we go again with the vicious cycle:

Pumping your body full of caffeine with coffee, tea, soda, or chocolate will jolt your adrenal glands and mimic a stress response. The acidity of caffeinated beverages can also disturb the lining of the intestinal tract and result in inflammation. Consuming large amounts of alcohol will damage the intestinal tract, upset your blood sugar levels, stress your liver, and ultimately act as a stimulant.

Eating more than a moderate amount of sugar will obviously distort your blood sugar, and since cortisol is the body's antidote to elevated insulin, it's likely that your cortisol levels will rise. If you eat a lot of sugar and fast foods, you're depriving the adrenal glands of the nutrients they need from fresh fruits and vegetables to function properly, since the adrenal glands require more vitamin C than any other tissue of the body.

You also stand a good chance of gaining weight, and as your weight increases, you're less likely to exercise. Exercise is very helpful in keeping your adrenal glands balanced, and it's a good way to get the stress of everyday life out of your system.

Another negative consequence of eating too much sugar or processed foods that convert easily to sugar is that it causes the pancreas to keep pumping out insulin, to the point where the over-secretion of insulin results in low blood sugar, or *hypoglycemia*. As the pancreas struggles desperately to keep the level of blood sugar normal in the face of a constant barrage of sugar, it can over-secrete insulin and pull too much sugar out of the bloodstream. The end result is low blood sugar and the further craving for sugar, which perpetuates the cycle over and over again.

As mentioned earlier, a pro-inflammatory diet is one that is so high in hydrogenated oils, trans-fatty acids, and saturated fats that it will increase levels of the inflammatory chemical prostaglandin-E2 (PG-E2) to the point where systemic inflammation occurs. And remember the rule: where there's inflammation, the body will secrete cortisol. PG-E2 is such a potent inflammatory chemical that it's the biological equivalent of pouring gasoline on a fire.

Omega-6 oils and saturated fats occur in nearly every form

of fast food; in processed foods such as crackers, cookies, donuts, and baked goods; and in anything made with corn oil. These oils are in the omega-6 class of fats, and they cause an increase in inflammatory chemicals. Since we all know by now what the body's response to inflammation is, we can expect a rise in cortisol along with all the potential problems that accompany it.

There is one last, very serious problem with a diet high in omega-6 fats as regards hormonal balance, and that is its effect on the actual *receptor sites* on every cell in the body.

Simplistically, receptor sites are like little fingers on the outer wall of a cell that are the doorways by which things get in and out of a cell. The hormones, as well as n*eurotransmitters* such as *serotonin* and *dopamine* (these are critical to regulating our mood and brain function as well as virtually every chemical a cell needs to function normally), need to be able to attach to specific receptor sites in order to enter the cell and affect cellular function.

These receptors are made of protein and are embedded in a fat membrane that makes up the outer wall of each cell. If the fat wall is soft (in neuroscience the terms used are *fluid* or *plastic*), then the neurotransmitters can easily dock on to the receptors. However, if the fat wall becomes hard and less fluid, the shape of the receptor site changes and the neurotransmitters cannot adequately attach to the receptors, with the result that the cell becomes impaired. The consequences of this situation on human health are enormous and can result in depression (serotonin deficiency), Parkinson's disease (dopamine deficiency), and any number of hormonal imbalances, because the hormones simply cannot communicate with the cells.

The scenarios I have been describing here are not uncommon and doctors' offices are filled with patients whose health problems are spiraling out of control. Since doctors are trained to treat specific symptoms with specific drugs, these patients can quickly find themselves on multiple medications for insomnia, depression, pain, and gastric upset that fail to address the causal factors of their health problems—namely intestinal tract inflammation, a pro-inflammatory diet, and cortisol imbalances. In the upcoming chapters, I'll show you how to accurately test your cortisol levels, resolve intestinal tract and systemic inflammation, restore hormonal balance, and get you on the road to regaining your health.

Richard Weinstein, D.C.

TESTING CORTISOL LEVELS

The Conditions for Murder are Met

If your health status resembles what I have been describing in the preceding chapters, then it's very probable that your cortisol levels are out of balance. If you're having trouble sleeping, find yourself craving sugar and/or salt, and you feel irritable and overwhelmed most of the time, then your cortisol levels are unstable. But it's not enough to assume that your cortisol levels are out of balance; we need to know **when** they are out of balance and by how much.

Fortunately, there is an easy and highly accurate way to find out just what your adrenal glands are doing throughout the day using a method known as salivary testing. Since hormones enter the saliva through passive diffusion of the soft tissue of the saliva glands, they can be tested by taking saliva samples at precise times of the day to see how well the adrenal glands are adapting to stress.

The National Aeronautics and Space Administration (NASA) has long been using salivary testing to measure the cortisol levels of its astronauts. One of the serious obstacles to lengthy space missions is the stress of confinement in a small capsule with seven other people for nine months, as would be the case during a trip to Mars. Astronauts who had spent several months aboard the space station Mir warned NASA years ago that the claustrophobic conditions could easily result in a homicide. One Russian cosmonaut, upon returning to Earth and commenting on the stress and tension of the mission, was quoted as saying, "The conditions for murder are met." So in an effort to avoid what would be a supremely embarrassing, "Houston, we have a problem" communiqué, NASA employs salivary cortisol testing.

NO WONDER YOU FEEL LIKE CRAP!

The Adrenal Stress Index

The saliva test for adrenal function is called the Adrenal Stress Index (ASI) test, and is done in the comfort of your home or workplace over the period of a single day. The test comprises four vials for the collection of saliva samples. Each vial is labeled with the time the sample should be collected, which is morning, noon, late afternoon (five to six P.M.), and midnight.

After collecting a sample in the appropriate vial, it's stored in the refrigerator; once all the samples have been taken, you ship them to the laboratory via overnight mail. There are laboratories that can evaluate these tests (see the Resource Guide at the end of book), and the one I use is Diagnos-Techs, Inc. The test results are sent back to your doctor with detailed graphs that chart your cortisol/DHEA levels and ratios.

The ASI test also measures blood sugar levels, intestinal tract inflammation, and the antibody *SIgA* that protects the intestinal tract and also detects any allergic reaction in the intestinal wall to wheat, rye, oat, and other grains that contain gluten. This can be very useful as a marker for intestinal tract inflammation and Candida infections.

In the previous chapters we went through the downward spiral of the adrenal glands' struggle to keep up with stress. The real value of the salivary test is that it will show us what **phase** of trouble the adrenal glands are in, as there are several. Unlike a blood test that simply measures the highs or lows of cortisol levels, the salivary test measures the **relationship** between cortisol and DHEA levels and can paint a clear picture of how well or how badly the adrenal glands are doing. This knowledge is important in determining the best course of treatment.

Briefly, the phases of adrenal gland function or malfunction, in descending order from fine, to bad, to worse, are:

1. Normally adapted to stress: the adrenals are coping well with normal levels of both cortisol and DHEA.

2. Adapted, with a slump in DHEA production: this means that the adrenal glands are having to make so much cortisol that they are not able to make as much DHEA.

3. Maladapted Phase I: signifies a further progression in which the adrenal glands are still able to make cortisol but the DHEA levels are becoming even lower.

4. Maladapted Phase II: this is where both the cortisol and DHEA levels are becoming low as the adrenal glands struggle to keep up with continued levels of stress or inflammation.

5. Non-adapted, low reserves: now the adrenal glands are not adapting to the need to make cortisol and DHEA, and the levels of both are falling lower.

6. High DHEA: this means the adrenal glands can no longer make cortisol but can still make some DHEA.

7. Adrenal fatigue: this is pretty much the end of the line as the adrenal glands can no longer make enough cortisol or DHEA; this is what we find in chronically ill patients.

Blood Tests Vs. Saliva Tests

Many doctors do not yet understand the importance of measuring cortisol levels, and those who do often rely on a blood test. Unfortunately, there are three problems in trying to assess cortisol levels in this manner.

The first problem is that a person's cortisol level may be fine during one part of the day but unbalanced during another part of the day. For example, it's not unusual for me to see an adrenal stress index test where the cortisol level is fine in the morning, too low in the afternoon, and then too high late at night. Any combination of these variances throughout the day can and do occur, so trying to accurately measure cortisol levels with a single blood sample taken at whatever time of the day you happen to see your doctor is not going to tell the whole story.

The second problem is that some people become so nervous in a doctor's office that their blood pressure goes up and causes inaccurate readings. This is known as *white coat syndrome*, and if it can elevate a person's blood pressure, then it will certainly elevate his or her cortisol levels and yield inaccurate results.

The third problem with using a blood test is that it will reflect the total hormone level and not what is called the *unbound bioactive fraction*, which is the actual hormone level as it affects cell function. In this way, blood-serum testing is not very reflective of what is really happening inside your body.

Since 1983, more than 2,500 scientific papers and research articles pertaining to salivary diagnostic testing have been published, yet salivary testing has still not come into mainstream medical practice. In addition to adrenal gland function, many other hormonal profiles (e.g., female hormone levels, both pre- and postmenopausal, as well as *testosterone*) can be tested using this method.

One of my goals in writing this book is to make salivary adrenal testing as routine as all the other diagnostic tests that patients take in their annual physical examinations. If your doctor is so concerned about your glucose and cholesterol levels, then why not be equally concerned about your cortisol levels? Should your doctor express no interest in checking your adrenal gland function, the Resource Guide at the end of the book will guide you to doctors who are familiar and competent in interpreting adrenal stress indexes and other salivary tests.

Richard Weinstein, D.C.

THE RELATIONSHIP OF CORTISOL TO OTHER DISEASES

The Missing Link

In the beginning of this book I gave you a virtual laundry list of diseases and disorders that can be caused by cortisol imbalance. Perhaps the reason you've chosen to read this book is because you have one of these health problems and either are hoping to better understand its causal factors or would like to learn other approaches to managing it. As an easy reference guide, I'm going to summarize each one of these disorders and explain the involvement of cortisol and DHEA imbalances.

Heart Disease

One way our bodies respond to stress is by constriction of the blood vessels in order to raise blood pressure and increase the delivery of oxygenated blood to our fight-or-flight muscles. Unfortunately, the continuous constriction of blood vessels due to chronic stress can result in damage and plaque buildup (this occurs because the constriction and increased blood pressure against the wall of the artery can cause the layers of the vessel to break down).

Your arteries have three layers, and the innermost one is very smooth, so that all the round blood cells can roll through the arteries quickly. The middle layer of the artery is sticky in order to hold the inner and outer layers together. The compromise in this wonderful design occurs where a larger artery divides to become smaller arteries. It's at this juncture that the increase in blood pressure, continually pounding away at this dividing point, weakens the inner wall and causes it to peel away.

As the inner layer becomes degraded, the middle, sticky layer becomes exposed. This allows the fats, starches, and calcium floating around in the bloodstream to adhere to its flypaper-like surface. Over a prolonged period of time this will result in the buildup of plaque found in heart disease and *atherosclerosis* (hardening of the arteries). As the plaque becomes thicker, it blocks the artery and restricts blood flow to the muscular wall of the heart. By choking off the flow of oxygenated blood, the cells of the heart muscle progressively die, and thus the stage is set for a heart attack.

We have been led to believe that heart disease is attributable to high-fat diets and elevated levels of cholesterol. However, this is not accurate, as shown by research done by physiologist Jay Kaplan of Bowman Gray Medical School. Kaplan has proved that social stress alone can cause atherosclerosis and high blood pressure in mice and primates and that this can occur even with a low-fat diet. So the real culprit is cortisol.

It's not only arterial plaques and restricted blood flow that can cause heart attacks, but also arterial spasms induced by strong emotional states, especially anger. Researchers at the University of North Carolina have published a study that finds a threefold increase in the frequency of heart attacks in people who are prone to fits of anger. This is related to the fact that cortisol constricts blood vessels.

Diabetes

Diabetes mellitus is the fourth leading cause of death in the United States, and it comes in two varieties.

The first type is *insulin-dependent* diabetes mellitus (IDDM), which refers to the inability of the cells of the pancreas to produce adequate amounts of insulin on demand. This type comprises only between five and ten percent of all diabetes cases and the major one risk factor is thought to be genetic. As the name implies, people with IDDM are dependent on insulin as a necessary part of their treatment. Depending on the severity of the diabetes, the insulin may be taken orally in pill form, or it may require injections to keep blood sugar levels stable.

The second type of diabetes is called *non-insulin-dependent* diabetes mellitus (NIDDM), and it affects the other ninety to ninety-five percent of diabetics. The number of people suffering from this type of diabetes is staggering, and the incidence of it has risen almost fifty percent since 1983. A stunning **8.3%** of Americans have this type of diabetes, and there is an average of 1.9 million new cases each year. In this type of diabetes, the pancreas is actually making insulin, but the cells have become desensitized, or resistant to the insulin.

Insulin resistance means that the receptor sites on the cell walls that are there to bind insulin to allow glucose to enter the cells have become resistant to the insulin. Being resistant to your own insulin is about the same as not producing insulin: either way, you cannot effectively utilize glucose. In an effort to correct this, your pancreas responds to the resistance by producing more insulin, and while this doesn't help in glucose utilization, it does seriously raise the level of triglycerides in your system, thereby increasing the risk of heart disease. To make matters worse, insulin signals the liver to make more cholesterol, so as the pancreas keeps secreting more insulin in response to your resistance, your cholesterol levels keep rising.

One of the principal functions of cortisol is to counteract the effects of insulin, because in fight-or-flight stress you don't want to store energy—you need to mobilize it immediately to meet life-threatening demands. One of the ways cortisol accomplishes this is by making your cells resistant to insulin, which for short-term stress management is appropriate. But when the cortisol level remains chronically elevated, it can become a factor in non-insulin-dependent diabetes mellitus, as long-term insulin resistance sets in and the pancreas struggles to produce ever-escalating quantities of insulin.

Amy originally came to see me for a very serious lower back problem, but during her course of treatment, she one day broke down crying. She had diabetes and had been on medication for five years, but when she saw her medical doctor the week before, he explained that if she could not keep her blood sugar levels consistently lower, she was likely to end up with damage to the arteries in her legs. Unfortunately, this can lead to gangrene and loss of limbs.

The problem in keeping her blood sugar numbers down was her uncontrollable craving for sugars and starchy foods. Even though she knew how much she was hurting herself by eating them, nothing could stop her from doing so. She felt horribly guilty about not being able stop eating the things that could actually kill her, and was at her wits' end.

*I explained to her that the problem she was having came from several factors that she didn't have a clue about and that it wasn't her fault that she couldn't stop eating sugars and starchy foods. First, her elevated cortisol was making it hard for her body to use the insulin medication she was taking, so her brain wasn't getting the sugar it needed to function properly. <u>This will cause such an intense craving for sugar that even though our rational mind tells us not to eat it, the brain literally commands us to eat it **anyway**.</u> As if this wasn't bad enough, Amy's negative emotion of guilt was causing an increase in inflammatory chemical in her blood that caused further elevations of cortisol, which only made her insulin levels worse. Another vicious cycle of stress.*

Amy responded very well to the 3R Program and in just three weeks all of her sugar cravings were gone and she was able to keep her blood sugar within a normal range.

Insomnia

In a properly functioning system, cortisol secretion follows a definite circadian rhythm, with the highest levels typically occurring at eight o'clock in the morning and progressively declining throughout the day. Since the function of cortisol is to create a state of alertness and arousal as a necessary response to stress, elevated levels of cortisol at night will obviously cause insomnia.

As discussed earlier, there are two types of insomnia—one where you can't fall asleep to begin with, and the other, more common one, in which you have no problem falling asleep but are awake again after three or four hours and have trouble getting **back** to sleep. Not being able to fall asleep easily is usually associated with blood sugar imbalances and high levels of cortisol at night when they should be very low. The inability to **stay** asleep is related to intestinal tract inflammation and the secretion of cortisol in the middle of the night as the body wants to repair connective tissue, realizes the intestinal tract is inflamed, and produces the cortisol in response to the inflammation.

Nearly everyone has experienced an episode of insomnia in his or her life because of an immediate stressor, such as worrying about an exam, a job interview, or some unpleasant situation that needs to be resolved. In the normal response to stress, these short-term episodes resolve as the stressful situation passes.

If the cause of the insomnia is psychological stress of a more serious or chronic nature, there is still every hope that with counseling, the use of better stress-management tools, or even just the passing of time, the issue will be resolved and the cortisol levels will return to normal.

Unfortunately, if the reason for the elevated cortisol levels is physiological, as in the case of inflammation, the insomnia will persist until the inflammation is resolved. We are then back to a vicious cycle in which the loss of sleep creates more stress, and—since cortisol inhibits the body's repair processes— this increase in stress can result in intestinal inflammation. To make matters worse, it's during sleep that the normal maintenance and repair processes occur; so if you aren't sleeping, you can't rebuild tissue effectively.

Often, insomnia sufferers will decide to enlist the aid of alcohol, especially if they're already experiencing pain in their joints or muscles. This only adds more fuel to the fire because alcohol will further degrade the intestinal lining, put an additional burden on the liver, and (since alcohol is technically a stimulant) it will contribute to the inability to successfully sleep through the night. Similarly, using one of the "p.m." preparations, which are a combination of anti-histamine and anti-inflammatory medications designed for nighttime use, will also further irritate the intestinal tract.

As is often the case with many of my patients, Donald came to me for treatment of one problem and ended up with having several other problems resolved. His reason for seeing me was chronic lower back pain, but during his consultation with me it turned out that he rarely slept through an entire night without waking up between 2:00 – 3:00AM and then found himself unable to get back to sleep for at least an hour. Many people who suffer from chronic pain have this problem because they take anti-inflammatory medications which inflame the intestinal tract, thus causing their body to secrete cortisol in the middle of the night in a futile attempt to resolve the inflammation. In Donald's case, the lack of sleep was also making him irritable and tired by mid-afternoon.

So while I was resolving Donald's lower back pain (this will be discussed in Chapter 7), I put him on the 3R Program and by the fourth week he was sleeping through the night. Even when he got up to go to the bathroom in the middle of the night, he was able to get back to sleep right away. The return of a normal sleep pattern also fixed the irritability and he was no longer tired during the day.

Depression

If you're a doctor, like myself, who is treating people with chronic pain and/or hormonal imbalances, then you're also going to see a lot of depressed people.

Alex came to see me for chronic, debilitating neck pain that kept him awake and prevented him taking part in many physical activites that he used to enjoy. He began feeling depressed over the previous four years and was clearly confused by this, because he thought he was doing a good job of adapting to his pain and limitations. What Alex didn't realize was that research proves that you cannot have pain without inflammation, and that all the pain medications he had been taking for so long were inflaming his intestinal tract and elevating his cortisol levels.

Richard Weinstein, D.C.

In addressing his neck pain, many factors had been missed, including showing him proper ergonomics and posture for reading and computer work, the need for cold compresses to heal his chronically weak ligaments, and gentle spinal manipulation to relieve pain and restore function (discussed in Chapter 7). However, it was the 3R Program that brought his cortisol levels down to where they weren't disturbing his brain chemistry and interfering with his ability to make and use serotonin, the neurotransmitter that makes us happy.

Well, if you're not already depressed by all this, let me show you why you could be.

People who suffer depression caused by imbalances in brain chemistry show hyperactive hypothalamic-pituitary-adrenal activity accompanied by increased levels of cortisol, as well as significantly higher morning and midnight salivary cortisol levels. There is also a great deal of scientific literature that discusses the correlation between fluctuating cortisol levels and daily mood swings. This goes a long way in explaining why you can feel pretty good during one part of the day, and then, for no apparent reason, your mood sinks and you're depressed. It also highlights the importance of the twenty-four-hour adrenal stress index salivary test to chart the cortisol circadian rhythm.

People suffering from depression are prone to further hypersecretion of cortisol when faced with recurrent or new stressors, meaning that they handle stress poorly. So here we are again, with a bad situation getting worse. If you're one of these people, you probably don't have a clue what is happening: there is really nothing occurring in the external factors of your life, such as your job, your relationship with your spouse, or your finances, that could account for you being so depressed. But you are.

Recent research tells us just how vicious this cycle can be, because negative emotions cause an increase in those nasty inflammatory *cytokines* (molecules that enable cells to communicate with each other, but are inflammatory most of the time). And as we all know by now, any increase in inflammation will bring about an increase in cortisol, and research studies show that people with depression **already** have increased cortisol levels. So the worse you feel emotionally, the further your cortisol levels rise, making you feel even more depressed.

In my clinical experience I have found that people will create almost any "reality" in an attempt to justify what they think or feel. So when—in an attempt to explain their depression—they decide to blame their spouse, kids, boss, coworkers, etc., serious problems can and will follow: it's called **looking for trouble**. This behavior will, of course, make the object of your blame react in ways that are bound to make you even more depressed, as in receiving your divorce papers or pink slip.

There is also another way in which intestinal tract inflammation and cortisol imbalances cause depression, and this is related to serotonin production. Serotonin, you may remember, is one of the neurotransmitter chemicals that makes us happy, and most antidepressant medications work by blocking the brain's ability to keep serotonin away from the cells that affect our mood.

The theory is that the more serotonin available to these brain cells, the less depressed you will be. While antidepressant drugs work for some people, this theory completely ignores the fact that the brain is responsible for synthesizing only **one percent** of the body's total serotonin production, while the other ninety-nine percent is synthesized in the intestinal tract. Since **ninety-nine percent** of all the body's neurotransmitters are made in the intestinal tract, it's easy to see how any number of brain chemical disorders can occur if the intestinal wall is inflamed and unable to make these chemicals that are vital to proper brain function.

Although this by no means discounts other causes of depression involving imbalances in brain chemistry or tragic circumstances, just understanding that one possible cause of your depression is a hormonal imbalance that can be tested for and treated can be very liberating, and it will take a lot of pressure off you and those around you.

Richard Weinstein, D.C.

PMS (Pre-Menstrual Syndrome) and Menopause

Because I find the phenomenon of hot flashes that occur with menopause so easy to correct, I get a lot of women referring their friends to me, since this can be a vexing problem that seems to defy treatment, especially if you don't want to run the risks associated with pharmaceutical hormonal replacement therapies.

Margie was a fifty-eight-year-old woman who was initially both sceptical and rather defiant about my ability to help with her hot flashes, from which she'd suffered every day and especially at night for the past two years. She woke several times a night and often had to change her nightgown because it was drenched in perspiration, and the flashes were triggered in the daytime whenever she became stressed or nervous—a serious problem when she had to give high-level presentations at work. Among the many reasons she was so sure I wasn't going to be able to help was because she had tried all manner of herbs and potions prescribed by Women's Health Centers, acupuncturists, and naturopaths that didn't work, and the fact that she'd suffered from severe PMS since her late 20's.

What was never factored into the equation of her hormonal problems was that in her late teens and early 20's she was an alcoholic and addicted to pain pills. While she was able to successfully recover from these addictions, her intestinal tract never did. The 3R Program addressed the inflamed intestinal tract, resolved her inflammation, and restored her hormonal balance to the point where the hot flashes resolved in five weeks, to her lasting joy and amazement.

PMS is so common that most women think it's just a normal part of having a monthly cycle during which they can expect all manner of symptoms including irritability, short-temperedness, multiple food cravings, emotionally oversensitivity, and depression.

The role of cortisol in PMS is due to the fact that the adrenal glands make *pregnenalone*, the substance necessary to make all the body's hormones. If the adrenal glands are too busy making cortisol, they'll just hog up the pregnenalone and there won't be enough left to make the proper amount of estrogen or *progesterone*. The end result of this imbalance in the normal ratio of these two hormones are the PMS symptoms.

Menopause is probably the single most misunderstood female hormone problem imaginable. Menopause should be absolutely nothing more than the end of a woman's monthly menstrual cycles, plain and simple, with no hot flashes, mood swings, or food cravings. All that is supposed to happen when the ovaries stop making hormones is that the adrenal glands take over and make an estrogen-like replacement hormone (*androstenedione*) for the rest of the woman's life. But just like what happens with PMS, if the adrenal glands are working to make cortisol because of excessive inflammation, then they won't have anything left with which to make the estrogen replacement hormone.

Now here comes the vicious cycle again: because estrogen acts in part to reduce inflammation, by not making any more estrogen (or the adrenal version of it), there is an increase in inflammatory chemicals in the bloodstream... So the adrenals produce more cortisol to try to reduce the inflammation. As a consequence, the chances of the adrenal glands making the replacement hormone just drop off the chart.

Sadly, menopause has created an entire pharmacopeia of hormone replacement therapies, bio-identical hormone madness, and herbal formulas of questionable value. By just taking a commonsense approach to restoring hormone balance, I find that resolving the symptoms attributed to the otherwise normal occurrence of menopause is a simple process. All that's necessary is to ensure that the adrenal glands can make the natural estrogen-like replacement hormone, and the "symptoms" subside.

Chronic Fatigue Syndrome

This syndrome is characterized by persistent or relapsing debilitating fatigue for at least six months, in the absence of any other definable medical diagnosis. Chronic Fatigue Syndrome patients exhibit low cortisol levels and adrenal insufficiency, meaning that their adrenal glands can no longer respond normally to stimulation from the pituitary gland messenger chemicals, and are in the fatigue phase of adrenal gland problems.

Richard Weinstein, D.C.

Symptoms of patients suffering from Chronic Fatigue Syndrome include depression, insomnia, low blood pressure, obesity, and the inability to cope with stress. The cortisol deficiency may also lead to impairment of the immune system, evidenced by an elevation in the concentration of certain antibodies in people with this syndrome.

Carmen was nearly certain that she was losing her mind: the rational part of her brain knew how important it was for her to function, yet the rest of her only wanted to lie down and do nothing. Her husband had been unemployed for over a year and it was up to her to support the family. She woke up tired, struggled to get through the day, and found herself craving sugar all the time. As someone who'd always taken pride in her good eating habits, she found this lack of control particularly infuriating. She simply couldn't make sense of what was happening to her, and, worse, was growing increasingly frightened and depressed about her ability to carry on like this.

Carmen's ASI test (Adrenal Stress Index) clearly showed that her adrenal gland function had burned out, that she had intestinal tract inflammation, a blood sugar imbalance, and also suffered from a Candida yeast overgrowth in her intestinal tract. How she managed to get to this sad place was through a combination of chronic stress and the long-term use of anti-inflammatory, over-the-counter ibuprofen for injuries she suffered in an automobile accident many years ago.

I treated Carmen with my 3R Program—<u>R</u>epair the intestinal tract, <u>R</u>esolve inflammation, <u>R</u>estore hormonal balance— supplemented by chiropractic treatment for her chronic pain from the automobile accident. A crucial part of her road to wellness was to help her understand that with her particular set of physical problems, it was completely natural for her to crave sugar and be depressed, and that she was neither "losing her mind", nor was she "a bad person who has no self-control." I also assured her that as her cortisol levels returned to normal and her intestinal tract inflammation resolved, she would (a) no longer crave sugar uncontrollably; (b) her energy level would gradually improve; and (c) her ability to think clearly would return. Sure enough, after twelve weeks she was fully back to normal.

NO WONDER YOU FEEL LIKE CRAP!

Weight Gain and Obesity

Stephanie was thirty-two when she came to see me for neck pain. She also expressed her frustration at not being able to lose the weight she gained since being pregnant three years previously. She had tried several different diet and exercise programs but nothing ever resulted in any weight loss.

Stephanie suffered multiple causes of stress from being a working single mom, and she had a fair share of stress in her relationships with men. She also had a typical profile of craving sugar and salt, mood swings, getting tired in the middle of the day, and PMS. I performed an ASI test and it reflected intestinal tract inflammation, as well as insulin and cortisol imbalances. Her case was even more challenging because she also had thyroid symptoms, and the thyroid gland regulates metabolism and the burning of calories.

So we did the 3R Program and while it took about six months to finally get everything balanced out, she did ultimately lose thirty pounds and has kept it off with no problem.

Unbalanced cortisol levels have been linked to obesity. Because cortisol affects so many systems in the body and will make you crave sugar, salt, and fat, this can occur in several different ways. To make matters worse, the foods that most often contain sugar, salt, and fat are usually high in inflammatory omega-6 oils, thus reinforcing the classic vicious cycle of elevated cortisol levels in response to inflammation.

First of all, many people use food as a means of reacting to stress. This will be discussed more comprehensively in Chapter 8, *The Not-So-Common Commonsense Diet*, but suffice it to say that certain foods represent emotional comfort for some people, and they will gravitate to those specific foods to achieve the desired emotional state. For example, if a Hostess Ding-Dong or a Snickers candy bar reminds you of a happy time in your childhood, you might use them to emotionally transport you away from your adult stresses.

As I mentioned earlier regarding diabetes, it's a fact that cortisol disrupts normal blood sugar levels due to its effect on insulin and by making the receptor site on cells resistant to insulin. The end result of not being able to get sugar into your cells, particularly those in your brain, is that your brain is going to demand you eat more sugar to feed it. Our brain requires a full third of all the sugar (glucose) that we consume, so you can see why this will easily cause a craving for sugar or carbohydrate-laden foods.

The overconsumption of carbohydrates is an excellent way to gain weight because whatever glucose your body can't use will be stored as fat. If you exercise a lot, you might be able to exhaust the glucose stored in your muscles to the extent that you will convert the fat cells back to glucose as you continue to exercise. However, there is no guarantee that exercise will do this because elevated cortisol levels can also cause another type of cell receptor site resistance, this time to a hormone called *leptin*.

Leptin, a hormone produced by fat cells, regulates fat storage and goes to the hypothalamus to reduce appetite. High cortisol levels and the high levels of insulin that cortisol causes make the hypothalamus cells resistant to leptin, so you don't know when to stop eating and are unable to burn fat properly. The result is weight gain and obesity.

The adrenal glands are also responsible for making a hormone called *aldosterone*, whose function is to regulate the minerals in our body. If however the adrenal glands are very busy making a lot of cortisol, they may not be able to make all the other hormones they're supposed to in adequate amounts. And without adequate aldosterone, you can become deficient in sodium and will crave salty foods to make up for it—and salty snack foods are high in inflammatory omega-6 oils.

If all this weren't bad enough, elevated cortisol levels makes us feel totally stressed out; and eating fat causes the brain to make *endorphins*, which in turn act as an opiate and make us feel much better. So craving foods that have a high fat content is one way to make yourself feel better. But these foods are usually also high in inflammatory omega-6 oils that increase cortisol production, which just results in your feeling all stressed out again. And since fats are very high in calories, you're certainly going to gain more weight.

So when you consider that at least fifty percent of Americans have internal inflammation which results in high levels of cortisol, and that cortisol causes us to crave sugar, salt, and fat, it's no wonder we're getting fatter and more obese. And that we feel like crap.

Immune System Disorders, Allergies, and Autoimmune Disease

As discussed in Chapter 2, both Cortisol and DHEA levels have a dramatic effect on the immune system. In an experiment designed to measure the effect of cortisol on the body's production of white blood cells (T-cells) by challenging it with tetanus toxins, oral administration of cortisol resulted in a thirty-eight percent decrease in T-cell production. Since the T-cells are involved in every immune response to any invading organism (e.g., bacteria and viruses), as well as interacting with other immune system cells, this is clearly very bad news.

Once again, the reason cortisol is so highly suppressive of your immune system is because your body doesn't **need** an immune system when it thinks the only agenda is survival. No doubt you may need your immune system to heal your wounds after you have successfully fought off a predator, but while you're stressed, cortisol will suppress your immune cell production. All this is great for short-term stress, but it can be disastrous in the long term.

The T-cells are produced in the bone marrow and mature in the thymus gland, and DHEA protects the thymus gland from the effects of cortisol, which is just another example of the way in which the body's miraculous system of checks and balances works to achieve homeostasis. It also helps explain why every person who is stressed doesn't necessarily get sick. The immune system only gets into trouble when the stress becomes chronic; the adrenal glands then go into the maladaptive phase, and the cortisol/DHEA ratios become compromised. It's when the immune system becomes chronically unbalanced that the stage is set for an autoimmune disease.

In any autoimmune disease, the immune system can no longer distinguish which cells belong to the body and which don't, and it begins to attack them as if they were foreign cells. The most common sequence of events goes like this:

- The intestinal tract, which actually is **seventy percent** of our entire immune system, becomes inflamed (current research states that an inflamed, leaky gut always occurs before any autoimmune disease)

- Cortisol is secreted in response to the inflammation.

- Cortisol suppresses the brain's chemical messengers that regulate the T-cells.

- Without these chemical messengers the T-cells are unable to distinguish the difference between foreign invading cells and the normal cells of your body.

- The T-cells launch an attack on your own cells. What determines which **type** of autoimmune disease you get, such as *lupus, multiple sclerosis, Hashimoto's thyroiditis,* or *rheumatoid arthritis*, is driven by genetics.

An example of how the cortisol/DHEA ratio participates in autoimmune disease is rheumatoid arthritis.
Rheumatoid arthritis is an autoimmune disease that can cause inflammation of the joints throughout the entire body. It affects approximately 2 million Americans and is considered to be a chronic disorder. It begins when the immune system attacks the synovial membrane between the joints that produces the lubrication that allows the joints to glide smoothly. As the inflammation progresses, the joint becomes swollen and painful. Eventually, the cartilage lining of the joint is destroyed, and the pain increases. People with rheumatoid arthritis also exhibit low serum-DHEA levels.

NO WONDER YOU FEEL LIKE CRAP!

Irritable Bowel Syndrome, Ulcers, and Colitis

One of the features of the human stress response, and the shift into the sympathetic nervous system mode that initiates it, is the shutting down of the parasympathetic nervous system, which is responsible for digestion. This makes a great deal of sense because when a tiger's chasing you, you need all your blood to go to your muscles rather than to the organs contending with a Whopper and fries. This is bound to create problems if the stress becomes prolonged, the two most obvious of which involve hydrochloric acid production and mucosal lining repair.

One of the pioneers of the physiology of stress was Hans Selye, who in the 1930s performed experiments on rats involving ovarian hormonal extracts. In one of the great ironies of science, Selye was a seriously clumsy individual who had difficultly injecting the rats because he kept dropping them, and therefore had to chase and retrieve them before he could continue his experiments—which of course proved to be a continuously stressful experience for the rats.

By the time Selye finished his experiment, he found that not only did the rats he injected with hormonal extracts have serious problems, but the control group he injected with only saltwater were also ill! As it turned out, both sets of rats had ulcers, debilitated immune systems, and enlarged adrenal glands. As a direct result of his ineptitude in handling rats and scaring the hell out of them, Selye went on to worldwide acclaim as a founder of the study of the human stress response.

The reason the rats had so many ulcers is because a part of the stress response is to shut down the body's repair mechanisms, which includes the mucosal lining of the digestive tract.

The enzymes that our bodies produce to break down the multitude of (sometimes bizarre) things that we put into our stomachs are very powerful. Hydrochloric acid, *pepsin*, and bile are strong chemicals that our bodies require to break down globs of proteins, carbohydrates, and fats. Since this (eating and digestion) is typically a thrice-daily process, there is a continuous need for the body to repair the mucosal lining that protects the gastrointestinal tract from these caustic enzymes. Unfortunately, high cortisol levels are excellent at inhibiting mucus secretion.

Being stressed out doesn't mean you stop eating; in fact, as we have seen, some people eat more when they are stressed. This constant onslaught of food and enzymatic activity, coupled with a breakdown of the stomach lining's repair process, results in patches of irritation and inflammation. As we all know by now, one of the body's responses to inflammation is to produce more cortisol; so around and around we go. If this cycle continues, the tissues can be degraded until an ulcer or hole develops.

Activation of the sympathetic nervous system, the part of the nervous system called upon in times of stress, will inhibit activity in the small intestines, where we absorb dietary nutrients, but will increase contractions in the large intestine, where waste products are processed and removed…Which accounts for the phenomenon of literally having the poop scared out of you at times of extreme perceived danger.

Chronic overstimulation of the large intestinal tract from stress will result in irritation and diarrhea, and the numerous medical diagnoses for these disorders include *colitis*, *irritable bowel syndrome (IBS)*, *spastic colon*, and *diverticulitis*. As is the case with the stomach and small intestinal tract, ulceration and bleeding can occur.

As a last thought regarding the effects of stress on the digestive tract, it's interesting to speculate on just what levels of dietary nutrients are actually being absorbed in people who are chronically stressed. Since the tiny, finger-shaped *villi* in the small intestine are responsible for nutrient absorption, and intestinal activity can be shut down during times of stress, it logically follows that chronically stressed people are unable to fully access food nutrients. This adds to their feeling unwell and contributes to their susceptibility to illness.

It gets worse. In a chronically inflamed intestinal tract, the villi may be damaged or even disappear as the intestinal lining is damaged. This is an overlooked but very important aspect of human nutrition, because it's not only what you eat, but also what you actually **absorb** into your bloodstream that matters. The best diet in the world isn't going to do you much good if the nutrients are literally going in one end and coming out the other without being broken down and absorbed.

When I was in my first year of practice, I encountered a middle-aged man suffering an acute case of lower back pain related to bending and lifting. He also had a chronic history of lower bowel problems which included alternating episodes of constipation and diarrhea as well as sharp bowel cramping. I took an X-ray of his lower spine, and to my horror saw three areas of abnormal bone density over the outside of his pelvic bone that looked a lot like cancer to me. Since I wanted to be absolutely certain of the diagnosis and didn't want to alarm him by prematurely mentioning the possibility of cancer, I called a radiologist at the local hospital for a consultation.

I was rather nervous when he put the X-ray on the light box because I was anticipating how terrible it was going to be to inform a patient that he had cancer. The radiologist looked at the film for several moments and burst out laughing. He informed me that while it was very reasonable for me to think that the white, dense shadows over the pelvic bone might be cancerous lesions, they were, in fact, calcium supplements that were passing through the intestinal tract completely undigested. At the time I took the X-ray, the calcium tablets were making their way down the descending colon, which lies in front of the pelvic bone.

At that early point in my career, I was so happy that I didn't have to tell this guy he had cancer that I totally missed the relevance of why he wasn't digesting his calcium supplements. What had happened was that his stress levels were so chronically elevated from the stress of his job and personal life, along with the more recent stress of intense back pain, that his intestinal tract had slowed down to the point where he could not properly digest what he was eating.

What I now know is that no diet or vitamin supplement program is going to help any of the conditions discussed in this chapter if you have an inflamed, debilitated intestinal tract or systemic inflammation that remains unresolved. For many people who suffer from chronic stress syndrome, intestinal tract inflammation may be the **single most important issue** to resolve, because if it persists, the cortisol and/or DHEA levels will remain unbalanced and perpetuate the digestive dysfunction. This results in the double whammy of having a not only a damaged digestive tract or insufficient numbers of villi for absorption of nutrients, but also a digestive tract working too slowly to produce the proper enzymes for digestion. Consequently, you will not be able to derive much benefit from the foods or vitamins necessary for good health.

Acid Reflux – Two Possible Causes

This is one of those cases that really makes me enjoy getting up in the morning and going to work.

Lillian was sent to me by the patient I told you about earlier with rheumatoid arthritis, as there was no obvious reason for her, or her parents, to think of seeing a chiropractor for acid reflux. A twelve-year-old girl who'd suffered from acid reflux for a year and a half, Lillian had received extensive medical care with no change in her symptoms. With no medications working, her doctors decided to put her on an antidepressant drug since they didn't know what else to do. This is when her parents put their foot down and decided this was not the path they wanted their daughter to go down.

As I was taking her case history and asking when does her acid reflux get better or worse, Lillian told me it always got worse if she was running or reaching over her head. On hearing this, a great big light went off in my head and I thought, "This girl has a serious psoas muscle spasm!" (Fully discussed in Chapter 7, Make the Pain Go Away*).*

The psoas muscles attach the lower back and pelvic girdle to the bottom of the shoulder girdle and enable us to lift each leg to walk, run, or climb steps; if they both contract, then you're bending over at the waist. The psoas muscles also attach beneath the diaphragm, where the esophagus meets the top of the stomach and the muscle sphincter that closes off the stomach from the esophagus. This sphincter is designed to close when food is in the stomach so the hydrochloric acid can't splash back up into the esophagus and burn it (the stomach has a protective lining for the acid and the esophagus does not).

So what Lillian was really telling me was that one of her psoas muscles was pulling on the diaphragm and preventing the sphincter from closing, so that the stomach acid splashed up. And it got worse if she really contracted the psoas muscle by running, or if she pulled on it by reaching up, because the muscle's tightness wanted to pull her forward as if bending over from the waist.

*When I examined her comparative psoas muscle tightness, she had the worst spasm I'd ever seen in my entire career! So I performed the psoas muscle release and showed her how to do it at home so she could keep it out of spasm herself. This **instantly** fixed her acid reflux because the sphincter could now close properly. The problem never came back.*

This next case is short and sweet and of a type which occurs frequently.

*An eighty-six-year-old man I'd treated over the past twenty-five years for various aches and pains decided to see me for acid reflux; we'd had a lot of success with his other problems, so he thought he would run this one by me. He'd been taking TUMS with every meal for the past four years, and I explained to him that his problem was not too much hydrochloric acid, but too **little**. So I gave him hydrochloric acid pills to take directly before each meal and told him to come back in five days to see if it was working. When he returned the acid reflux was completely gone and he also felt more energetic because now he was properly digesting his food.*

Many cases of acid reflux are poorly diagnosed and—even worse—treated incorrectly. The common perception is that somehow your stomach, for no obvious reason, has decided to produce too much hydrochloric acid, and that acid is causing an irritation of the lining of your stomach. This concept ignores the fact that the stomach has a protective lining of glycerin which is impervious to hydrochloric acid.

There are two better reasons why you may be suffering from acid reflux, commonly known as heartburn.

The first is that (as in the example above) you're actually producing too **little** hydrochloric acid because cortisol is inhibiting your pituitary gland from secreting a hormone called *gastrin*. This hormone tells your stomach cells to produce hydrochloric acid when you start eating. If you don't have enough acid in your stomach, the proteins you eat will literally stick to the wall of your stomach, putrefy, and form *pyruvic acid*, against which your stomach has no protection. The carbohydrates you eat will also not digest properly and will ferment, causing a sour sensation. The standard medical approach to this situation is to use drugs that block all acids, hydrochloric and pyruvic... Which begs the question of just how are you supposed to digest any of your food?

Keep in mind that if the mass of food in your stomach isn't acidic enough when it passes into the small intestinal tract, it won't trigger production of the other necessary enzymes in the liver and pancreas. This means you'll have a lump of poorly digested food in there that can't be broken down into nutrients, and it will create toxins that can cause intestinal tract inflammation. It also means that the pancreas can become dysfunctional and not secrete adequate amounts of insulin, leading to weight gain, obesity, and diabetes.

Another possible cause of acid reflux is an *H. pylori* infection in the stomach, which can be easily tested for and treated with antibiotics. Of course, after the antibiotic you need to take a *probiotic* formula of beneficial bacteria to replace the ones that the antibiotic killed off.

Thyroid Disorders

The suppression of thyroid function caused by high levels of cortisol leads to hypothyroidism (low thyroid function) and related illnesses. In such cases, there are decreased serum-DHEA levels as well.

The thyroid gland operates through a feedback loop, just like our earlier thermostat and furnace example, in which the pituitary gland secretes various hormones which prompt hormone production in the thyroid. But since twenty percent of thyroid hormone is activated in the intestinal wall, if the intestinal tract is inflamed and its function compromised, twenty percent of thyroid hormone may be lost.

The symptoms of hypothyroidism are fatigue, low blood sugar, chronic infections, obesity (are you beginning to see a pattern here regarding the effects of cortisol imbalance?), intolerance to cold, muscle weakness, and constipation.

Martha was thirty-five years old when she came to see me with a host of thyroid symptoms that included bloating after eating, constipation, cold hands and feet, depression, fatigue, insomnia, sugar cravings, and an inability to lose weight even though she exercised five times a week.

She first began having some of these thyroid symptoms in her early twenties but they became noticeably worse after a stressful and failed marriage. I put her on my 3R Program and recommended changes in her diet to include more protein, especially at breakfast, and to dramatically reduce her grain consumption. In addition to the usual supplements in the 3R Program I also put her on L-tyrosine *to support her ability to make thyroid hormone. After one month she was sleeping better and didn't need to take Ambien; the bloating and constipation were gone, she had no sugar cravings, and her energy was improving. After four months she was sleeping fine, her energy was good, her depression was gone, and she had lost four pounds. In another six weeks she was doing fine with no symptoms, and was able to lose a pound a week consistently.*

Fibromyalgia

Fibromyalgia is a disorder that began to gain notoriety in the mid-1980s and was initially viewed with scorn by the mainstream medical establishment because of its multiple symptomatology. As with chronic fatigue syndrome, it was given no credence, and people suffering with it were considered to be psychosomatic whiners with "yuppie flu." Today fibromyalgia is seriously regarded as an autoimmune disease in which the T-cells attack the muscles and tendons. When you consider the other symptoms of fibromyalgia, such as irritable bowel, insomnia and fatigue, depression, and loss of concentration, it's easy to see the sequence I have previously outlined as the basis for autoimmune disease at work here.

Richard Weinstein, D.C.

Memory Loss, Dementia, and Clarity of Thought

Karen was literally at her wits' end. At forty-nine she was no longer always able to remember whom she'd talked to in business meetings or sometimes what the meetings were even about, which was a serious problem when she was the one in charge of the meetings in the first place. Besides being frustrating, it was also flat-out frightening to think she was clearly heading towards some form of dementia or Alzheimer's disease.

Of course, stress was a major cause. The reason her stress levels were so high was (i) a very demanding job in which thousands of people were affected by her decisions; (ii) raising four children with almost no help from her husband; and (iii) poor eating habits. Put those factors all together and it caused her cortisol levels to become chronically high. In her case, the cortisol was progressively killing the brain cells that retain memories. And as vicious cycles go, well… The fear of losing her memory, mental capabilities, and possibly her job only worsened her stress and cortisol levels.

The 3R Program rebalanced Karen's cortisol levels, and I put a special emphasis on the supplements that would support cognitive function, such as omega-3 oils and Cytozyme PT/HPT *(discussed in Chapter 6,* Resolving Cortisol Imbalances*). I also helped to put together a better diet that included eggs, which she was afraid to eat due to the foolish cholesterol scare that eggs will kill you. Besides being one of the best complete sources of protein, eggs are very high in* acetylcholine, *which is the brain chemical necessary to make memories in the brain. Karen now has no problems with her memory or recall capabilities.*

The reason I wrote that it's important to understand some of the brain structures that deal with stress (such as the hypothalamus) is because of what happens to them when there is a cortisol imbalance, and how dramatically that can impact our health. It's terribly sad to see someone in otherwise reasonable health slip into dementia and memory loss, a condition from which there is no hope of return.

In Chapter 2, I described how the body orchestrates its response to stress using the example of the thermostat and furnace in your home, and that when the stress was successfully resolved, cortisol would go back up to the hypothalamus and shut the stress response off. This works just fine for short-term stress, as the cells of the hypothalamus are extremely sensitive to cortisol; but with long-term stress, cortisol can kill these cells. The problem is that memories, especially short-term ones, are made and stored in the hypothalamus. So, sure, you can remember what you did when you were twenty years old, you just can't remember what you had for dinner or the last time your kids visited you. As this progresses, even conscious awareness of who and where you are begins to collapse.

Our ability to think clearly and concentrate relies on two hormones, epinephrine and norepinephrine, both made by the adrenal glands and one also made by the thyroid. Since the adrenal glands can only do so much at any one time, if they're busy making cortisol because you have so much internal inflammation, they may not be able to make these other hormones. Add to this the fact that cortisol can cause thyroid dysfunction, and now maybe you can't make **any** of the hormones necessary for clear thinking and concentration. In thyroid patients this symptom is called, "brain fog."

Asthma

High cortisol levels relate directly to the inability to make epinephrine and norepinephrine as described above because these two hormones cause the bronchial tubes in your lungs to stay open and relaxed. When you look at the ingredients of most inhalers for asthma sufferers, you will note that these hormones are the active substances. There is also a condition known as *exercise induced asthma*, which is what happens when exercise raises the cortisol level and then there is not enough epinephrine or norepinephrine being made.

Jeanine originally came to see me for chronic episodes of neck and lower back problems, but her history included asthma since her early teens and she was using pharmaceutical inhalers to relieve her asthma symptoms. The 3R Program restored her hormone balance of epinephrine and norepinephrine and resolved her asthma. However, what she now finds interesting is that the asthma only comes back when her stress levels get too high. This lets her know that it's time to address whatever it is that's causing her to be stressed, and also reminds her that it's time to take the adrenal supplement (discussed in Chapter 6, Resolving Cortisol Imbalances*) that will lower her cortisol and allow her to make enough of the other hormones to stop the asthma.*

High Cholesterol

I want to throw the issue of high cholesterol into all this because it's so poorly understood and almost everyone has become convinced by their doctor that it's a big deal and will lead to heart disease, stoke, and diabetes. This is not exactly true, but it's a great way to scare people into taking statin drugs to reduce cholesterol, which we'll get into a bit later. The importance of high cholesterol is that it's caused by high levels of cortisol, and is, in fact, a **symptom** of high cortisol. So simply lowering the cholesterol and thinking you have reduced your risk of heart disease and diabetes is foolish.

The truth about cholesterol is that it's not made from the fat you eat; it's made in your liver from the sugars and carbohydrates you eat. Reducing the fat in your diet has nothing to do with lowering your cholesterol. Here's how cholesterol is really made:

- You eat sugars and carbohydrates.

- Once they reach your intestinal tract, insulin binds to the carbohydrates and carries them to your liver.

- The liver uses enzymes to turn the carbohydrates first into usable glucose, then into storable glycogen.

- Finally, what's left becomes cholesterol and triglycerides.

There are two factors that will cause too much cholesterol and triglycerides to be made.

The first is a diet that is too high in the bad carbohydrates that come with eating fast food and processed foods, because these simply supply more sugars and carbohydrates than your body needs, and your liver has no choice but to turn the excess into cholesterol. But the second and most significant problem is that these bad carbohydrates are also high in the inflammatory omega-6 oils, and that causes an increase in cortisol. Since cortisol makes you unable to use insulin properly (remember the fight-or-flight process?) and this in turn renders the liver unable to convert the carbohydrates into glucose and glycogen as it should, it turns them into cholesterol and triglycerides instead as a way of storing all this excess sugar.

This is an excellent way to become diabetic.

Cholesterol is absolutely necessary in making the protective lining for your nerves. Your brain is made up of a lot of cholesterol. And every single hormone your body makes starts with a substance made from cholesterol. So where's the problem and what's the big deal about it? The cholesterol isn't the problem, it's the symptom: the reason it's high is because high levels of cortisol make you unable to use your own insulin. It's the cortisol that causes this, and as you now know, it's really the cortisol that causes high blood pressure, heart disease, and diabetes. The high cholesterol is really just an indicator that all this is going on. And though the pharmaceutical industry doesn't have any drugs they can sell you to lower cortisol, they have plenty to lower cholesterol.

The pharmaceutical industry has drugs like Crestor, Lipitor, and Mevacor, and, at $35 billion dollars a year, these statin drugs are the highest-selling drugs in the world. American doctors have been sold on prescribing these drugs based on a single, seriously flawed study done in 1980 called JUPITER. The respected *Archives of Internal Medicine* reports that on the basis of this one study, millions of people have been put on these statin drugs that reduce your risk of heart disease by just **one percent**. That's it–only **one percent**, in a double blind study where one group was given a statin drug and the other group a placebo. Worse, it turns out that the drug company paid for the study and that nine of the fourteen authors of the JUPITER study were financially tied to the drug company.

The side-effects of statin drugs include memory loss, muscle and joint pain, liver dysfunction, stomach pain and diarrhea, headaches, fatigue, irritability, erectile dysfunction (don't worry, they have other drugs for that), and kidney failure. So to put this in its proper perspective, you end up on a statin drug that will lower your cholesterol but does nothing about the high levels of cortisol causing the high cholesterol—and you're still at risk of dying from heart disease and diabetes.

So far we have journeyed down a road of stress, disease, and despair, where the interaction between adrenal hormone imbalances and inflammation can result in one health problem after another. Now it's time to explore the 3R Program and how to get out of this mess, <u>R</u>epair your intestinal tract, <u>R</u>esolve the inflammation, and <u>R</u>estore your hormonal imbalance, so that you can, hopefully, live happily ever after.

RESOLVING CORTISOL IMBALANCES – THE 3R PROGRAM

A Plan That's Easy to Follow and to Swallow

To resolve these dangerous cortisol imbalances, I use my 3R Program:

Repair the intestinal tract, Resolve inflammation, and Restore hormonal balance

… And trust me that until you get the first two Rs managed, you will never get the hormones to balance.

Relevant Symptoms of Cortisol Imbalance

Insomnia

Difficulty in falling asleep usually indicates low blood sugar due to cortisol suppression of insulin. If you wake up in the middle of the night and have trouble falling back to sleep, this disturbance is due to an abnormal elevation of cortisol usually in response to an inflamed intestinal tract, and the cortisol causes alertness.

Depression/Anger/Anxiety/Moodiness

Any of these symptoms occurring without reasonable provocation (the house hasn't burned down, you didn't lose your job, no loved ones are ill or have died, all your retirement plan isn't invested in Florida swamp land) indicates that the adrenals are hyperfunctioning.

Sugar, Salt, and Chocolate Cravings

The suppression of insulin and interference with carbohydrate metabolism caused by high cortisol leads to cravings for sugar. Salt cravings are the result of a weakness in the adrenal glands' ability to manage the sodium-potassium pump that maintains the body's mineral content and the leakage of sodium out of the body. Do you crave chocolate? This is also a sodium-potassium pump problem, but this time it's magnesium that is leaking out, and chocolate is very high in magnesium.

Fatigue

Feeling tired all or most of the time, and normal activities seem like too much of an effort to either start or finish. This lack of vitality would be caused by adrenal hypofunction and insufficient cortisol and DHEA. It could also be related to cortisol's effect on thyroid function, or the intestinal tract being too inflamed to activate the twenty percent of thyroid hormone it's supposed to.

Low Libido

If you're a man, and your sex life can be described by the term "down and out;" or if you're a woman, and your attitude toward sex can be best described by "not that again"? This weak libido can be due to either adrenal hyper- or hypofunction, and the ASI (Adrenal Stress Index) will reveal the problem.

Fluctuating Energy Levels

Your energy level is generally good for the first part of the day but then it slumps either after lunch or around three or four o'clock in the afternoon. This fluctuation is the result of insulin resistance, which occurs when cortisol inhibits glucose from entering cells: the outcome is low energy and fatigue.

Craving Sugar After Dinner

Your appetite seem relatively normal for most of the day until you eat dinner, after which you obsessively eat anything you can get your hands on. This is another example of an unbalanced relationship between cortisol and blood sugar levels.

Cold Extremities and Inabilty To Lose Weight

Your hands and feet, or perhaps your entire body, feel cold most of the time even if the outside temperature is warm, or you're gaining weight even though you're not overeating. This would be indicative of a decrease in thyroid function that may be related to either adrenal and/or pituitary dysfunction.

Factors in Assessing the Risk of Intestinal Tract Inflammation

- Have you ever taken or do you still take NSAIDs frequently? In a similar vein, have you taken prednisone or any other cortisone drug for a prolonged period of time?

- Have you ever been on long-term antibiotic therapy, even as long ago as your childhood ear infections?

- Do you consume caffeinated beverages, and if so, which ones (coffee, tea, soda), in what quantities, and how frequently?

- Do you drink alcohol, and if so, what type, in what quantities, and how often?

- Do you frequently experience intestinal bloating after eating, have a lot of flatulence, or feel like you have trouble digesting your food?

- Do you have either constipation or diarrhea frequently, or else alternate between the two?

By piecing together these cortisol imbalance risk factors as indicated by your symptoms and with the results of the ASI, your doctor should be able to start you on the road to recovery. Again, it's important to remember that the hormonal system is exquisitely complex, and sometimes the nutritional supplements that work for one person will not always have the same effect on another.

Before We get Started – The Critical Importance of Healthy Receptor Sites

The receptor sites on cell membranes provide a perfect example of just how challenging the hormonal system can be. Remember, every cell in the body has receptor sites on its outer membrane wall, and these receptor sites are like little keyholes that are specific to particular chemical keys that attach themselves to the sites. These chemical keys can be nutrients, neurotransmitters, or hormones; and using this mechanism, the cell is able to selectively decide which chemicals go in and which go out, and what enzyme functions will occur.

The number of receptor sites for any specific hormone changes not only from day to day but minute by minute! Obviously, for hormones to work properly, there must be an adequate number of receptor sites available, and if these sites are compromised for any reason, then hormonal function will be equally compromised. This may be one explanation for why one person who has a good number of receptor sites available will improve more rapidly than another person whose receptor sites are diminished.

As we saw in previous chapters, a major factor in receptor site function is how soft the outer fat part of the membrane is. The receptor sites are made of protein and embedded in the fatty membrane; and the softness of the fat (lipid) wall is what determines the sensitivity, function, and number of receptor sites.

Diets that are high in trans fats and omega-6 oils (common in most processed foods and certainly fast/junk foods) cause the lipid membrane to become stiff and reduce receptor site function. Diets that are high in omega-3 oils promote membrane function. This again points to the importance of diet in resolving cortisol imbalances far beyond the obvious effects of caffeine and sugar, because if the receptor sites are not able to adequately bind neurotransmitters and hormones, the cell cannot function at its optimal level.

So a critical factor in your ability to get well is to have the receptor sites working well. If they're not, all the vitamin supplements in the world won't help you because those vitamins and nutrients can't get inside the cell where they're needed.

Repairing the Intestinal Tract: Glutamine

If the ASI test reveals intestinal tract inflammation, then treatment must begin with resolving that inflammation. I can't overstate how important this is, because no other therapy will have a meaningful long-term effect if the inflammation isn't addressed.

As an example, you can take all manner of adrenal supplements or prescription Diflucan or nystatin for Candida infections, but unresolved intestinal inflammation will still cause the adrenal glands to produce cortisol as an anti-inflammatory hormone, and you will eventually enter the vicious cycle of inflammation—increased cortisol production, which will cause continued inflammation, which will cause further cortisol production, and so on.

Here's an analogy: consider a patch of really bad soil that is weed-infested. You spray it heavily with weed killer, but then neglect to fix the soil. So the ground still isn't healthy enough for anything but weeds... And given just a little time, the weeds are going to grow back (as will the Candida in an unrepaired intestinal tract), and you're back to where you started.

A recent fad in the vitamin supplement world has people taking lots of probiotic beneficial bacteria thinking these are going to fix their digestive problems and improve their health. Just like the weed and soil example, the same problem comes up, except this time we will try to grow grass instead of kill weeds. So you still have the same lousy plot of soil (your inflamed intestinal tract) and now you're going to plant lots of good quality grass seeds (the probiotics) and expect them to grow and flourish. Not very likely.

Fortunately, I have a simple and logical sequence for you to follow in order to get well.

Resolving intestinal tract inflammation is the easiest part of the program. The intestinal tract can usually be repaired in as little as six to eight weeks by simply taking 1,500 mg of the amino acid *glutamine* twice a day on an empty stomach. Glutamine is one of the amino acids we get from eating protein, and there is abundant research that proves that glutamine plays a role in muscle formation, liver, kidney, and immune system function, and *antioxidant* production. There are no known side effects to taking glutamine, except for the rare occurrence of constipation if there is too little water and fiber in the diet. Glutamine is easy to find in any vitamin or health food store, where it's sold as L-glutamine (the "L" simply designates its molecular structure).

Back in 1978, a pharmacologist at the NIH (National Institutes of Health) named Herbert Windmueller discovered that glutamine was the major fuel used by the cells of the intestinal tract, and that glutamine depletion resulted in cell death. Since then, there have been numerous research studies that prove the effectiveness of glutamine in repairing the lining of the intestinal tract, restoring the normal tissue barriers in the intestinal wall (the little pinholes that result in leaky gut syndrome), and improving the intestinal immune function.

One of the most important research studies regarding glutamine was published in 1976 by Japanese scientists who induced ulcers in rats by giving them NSAIDs (aspirin, in this case). Two groups of rats were given the same amount of aspirin, but one group was also given L-glutamine. The administration of glutamine totally prevented the occurrence of ulcers in the rats.

I find it interesting—and very disturbing—that while glutamine is the most commonly used antiulcer drug in all of Asia, it's virtually unknown and unused in this country. And yet there are numerous prescription and over-the-counter medications used to treat ulcers in the United States that have several negative side effects. Remember, ours is a nation that has **16,500 deaths a year** from prescription NSAIDs due to intestinal tract bleeding, and these deaths could, for the most part, be prevented by simply taking glutamine (I recommend 1,500 mg) approximately one hour prior to taking the NSAIDs.

Glutamine must be taken on an empty stomach (i.e., no other protein eaten in the previous ninety minutes) to be clinically useful. The reason for this is that when you eat and digest protein, the glutamine has to compete for absorption, and it's therefore impossible to predict how much glutamine will be absorbed. By taking the glutamine without any proteins, we can be sure the body will get a good clinical dose.

The easiest way to take glutamine is on getting up in the morning, because your stomach is certainly empty at that time, and then just not eat protein for at least half an hour; then take it again at bedtime, assuming it's been over an hour and a half since you had dinner and you haven't eaten any protein since then. This is as easy as placing the bottle of glutamine on the nightstand next to your bed so that when you wake up and go to sleep, it's right there waiting for you. Alternatively, you can take the glutamine thirty minutes before eating a meal with protein, such as when you get home from work (assuming you're not going to eat for the next half an hour).

Glutamine is inexpensive and is available in capsules that usually contain 500 mg of L-glutamine, so a 1,500 mg dose would mean three capsules. You may also find it in 1,500 mg caps, so you can just take one in the morning and one at night. For people who have trouble swallowing pills, it also comes in a powder form.

Although I've seen several research articles that discuss much larger doses, in my clinical experience 1,500 mg twice a day is almost always enough to repair the intestinal tract in six to eight weeks, as long as the patient is not taking NSAIDs, drinking a lot of caffeine (more than two 6-ounce cups a day), drinking a lot of alcohol (more than two drinks a day), or drinking sodas that contain phosphoric acid (**zero** a day, because soda is **garbage**, plain and simple, and you'll hear more about this later). And if the patient is mixing all these factors together so that there are two cups of coffee, two sodas, two alcoholic beverages, and a couple of NSAIDs thrown in on a daily basis, forget about it!

Unless the patient is so seriously ill that there's no room for compromise, my approach is to ask my patients to decide which one of their vices is most important to them and to choose which ones they'll give up in order to get well.

Other Nutrition Supplements for Intestinal Tract Repair: Soluble and Insoluble Fiber

Soluble and insoluble fiber is found in vegetables and is very important in intestinal tract health and stability. Soluble fiber dissolves in water and insoluble doesn't, and as such they perform different functions in the gut. While the Dietary Guidelines for Americans recommend twenty-five grams of fiber per day for women and thirty-eight grams for men, most Americans get only fifteen grams, or half as much as they should be eating.

Soluble fiber attracts water and form a protective gel on the intestinal tract wall which has the important function of slowing down the rate at which sugar is released into the bloodstream. This is helpful in reducing insulin sensitivity and lowering cholesterol, since, as discussed earlier, both are the result of too much available sugar. It also helps to make you feel full, which can help with regulating food intake. Lastly, the protective gel is helpful in stabilizing leaky gut syndrome. Sources of soluble fiber are psyllium, guar gum, apples, pears, oranges, celery, carrots, and nuts.

Psyllium and guar gum can be bought in vitamin and health foods stores either as capsules or in powdered form. While it is obviously desirable to get dietary fiber through eating the required amount of vegetables, you can supplement your fiber intake by using either of these two. For example, a tablespoon of psyllium powder equals 6.7 grams of fiber, so two servings a day (morning and night) along with eating vegetables can really help you achieve the required amount of fiber. Most patients find the capsules easier to swallow, but this is a personal choice.

Insoluble fiber doesn't dissolve in water and passes through the intestinal tract undigested, so it adds bulk to the diet and helps with bowel movement regularity, thus removing toxins from the system. Sources of insoluble fiber include cabbage, onions, broccoli, zucchini, tomatoes, and cucumbers.

Killing the Candida Infection with Oregano Oil

It would be hard to find a condition so mistakenly treated by people trying to get healthy than Candida. They try the Candida diet and eliminate all sugars in an attempt to starve out the little buggers. Or they take probiotics and think they can repopulate their intestinal tract with the good bacteria in hopes of crowding out the Candida yeast population. Or they try oregano oil or other supplements to try to kill it.

The only problem is that this is completely ass backwards.

Julie entered my office with not only a shopping list of hormonal disorders but also carrying a big shopping bag filled with must have been twenty different vitamin supplements. She was on a lifelong quest to kill the Candida she had been battling for years, with the Candida winning every time. While she certainly had a Candida yeast infection or overgrowth which caused her to crave sugar and resulted in blood sugar imbalances (among various hormonal problems), her approach to the war was doomed to failure.

*The Candida infection is an **effect** of intestinal tract inflammation, not a **cause** of it, and it flourishes simply because the inflamed intestinal* *tissue is no longer a hospitable place for the other beneficial bacteria to live—so the Candida just takes over. Unless the intestinal tract is repaired first, it's pointless to keep trying to kill the Candida, because it will always come back.*

I put Julie on my 3R Program, and after six weeks of repairing the intestinal tract, we then went about the business of killing the Candida yeast, with complete success. Her sugar cravings also went away, which was an important step in getting her other hormones to balance out.

After taking the L-glutamine for six to eight weeks, it's now time to go about resolving a Candida overgrowth and also getting rid of other unwanted microbes in your intestinal tract. This doesn't mean you stop taking the L-glutamine, because it'll still continue to repair the intestinal tract; it just means it's probably safe to kill these microbes without the risk of them leaking out of the intestinal wall, since the L-glutamine has now fixed the leaky gut syndrome.

Science is making rapid progress in unlocking nature's secrets as regards plants and foodstuffs that provide more than just nutrients. One promising field of study concerns the variety of spices that have been used for centuries to add zest to a wide range of foods.

Long before the advent of refrigeration it was recognized that herbs and spices could slow down food spoilage through natural antimicrobial activity. Recent studies have focused on the effects of spices and their associated oils on food-borne organisms in the context of food safety and spoilage.

In the event the patient has an intestinal Candida Albicans infection, I use sustained-release emulsified oregano oil, which can be very effective in eradicating the yeast. An analysis of oregano reveals that its oil contains two antioxidant compounds that are effective in killing fungi and yeasts.

Biotics Research makes a product called ADP, in which they have microemulsified the oregano oil, thereby dramatically increasing its effective surface area, and then applied a sustained-release mechanism to it. The combined effect of microemulsification and sustained release is that it enhances the intestinal exposure to the oregano oil and thus its ability to eradicate the yeast.

Apex Energetics makes a supplement called MYCO-ZYME which also contains an extract of oregano oil and other herbal compounds for the removal of yeast and bacterial pathogens.

Oregano oil **can** be found in vitamin and health food stores, but I prefer using a pill form as the liquid oil is quite strong and sometimes hard to get down. However, I want you to be able to use nutritional supplements easily available in vitamin and health food stores and get started in the right direction on your own if you choose to. If you buy an oregano oil other than those from the manufactures listed above, simply follow the directions on the label.

Probiotics

Probiotic supplements contain multiple strains of beneficial bacteria that are necessary for the intestinal tract to function properly. Now that the intestinal tract is repaired and can provide a nice home for these friendly microbes to live in, it's time to start taking the probiotics. All vitamin stores sell these and you simply need to find one that has multiple bacterial strains and not only lactobacillus and acidophilus. Take them as recommended on the label.

Glutathione

Glutathione, a combination of three amino acids (*cysteine, glycine,* and *glutamate*), is the body's most powerful scavenger antioxidant, which means that it neutralizes *free radicals* which can destroy healthy tissue. Glutathione also helps to inhibit the production of the pro-inflammatory cytokines that occur with intestinal tract inflammation. Over the past five years, glutathione has become increasingly better understood as one of the major factors in longevity, and explains how someone with a terrible diet who drinks alcohol and smokes cigarettes can outlive someone with a great diet and clean lifestyle.

This is because of the genetic 'luck' factor in how much glutathione your body makes from the proteins you eat. If you're lucky, you have the genetic ability to combine the three amino acids that form glutathione when you eat protein. If, on the other hand, you're unlucky, you could be eating lots of good protein but lack the ability to make much glutathione out of it, in which case your ability to keep your immune system strong and remove dangerous chemicals from your body will be compromised.

It's seriously important to understand that you **cannot** take glutathione pills to increase your glutathione levels! If you can't genetically combine the three amino acids that form glutathione from the protein you eat, you'll still have the same problem taking it in pill form. The problem is that the glutathione pill is, after all, nothing more than the three amino acid proteins. Once your stomach extracts the three separate amino acids in the pill, your intestinal tract still has to assemble them into glutathione, just as it would any other form of protein. So either you're genetically lucky and you'll make glutathione out of any ingested protein… or you won't, in varying degrees.

Fortunately, there are a few ways to either help the process along, or to actually get glutathione into your system.

The single best way is to use an Apex product called Oxicell, which is a glutathione cream you apply to your skin, from which it goes directly into your bloodstream.

If you don't have access to a doctor who can give you Oxicell (please refer to the Resource Guide at the end of the book to see if you can find one in your area who practices Functional Medicine), the next way to help increase your glutathione levels is by taking a combination of *alpha lipoic acid* (250 mg) and *acetyl-l carnitine* (500 mg) daily. The benefits of this supplement combination were demonstrated in three research studies in which rats given these two supplements lived twice as long as rats in the control group because the supplements helped raise glutathione levels.

Further benefits can be obtained by taking *curcumin* (turmeric root extract) at 500 mg a day, as this also helps the body make glutathione.

Resolving Systemic Inflammation

Omega-3 oils

As I'll discuss in Chapter 8, systemic inflammation, i.e., elevated levels of inflammatory chemicals circulating throughout the body, can best be controlled by avoiding hydrogenated oils, fast foods, fried foods, baked goods, and processed foods that contain omega-6 oils. Supplements containing omega-3 oil from fish sources significantly reduce inflammation and are widely available at vitamin stores, drugstores, and even supermarkets.

Make sure it's a good-quality oil and preferably one whose label says that it's pharmaceutical grade. A good-quality omega-3 oil will be screened for mercury, pesticides, and other toxins, and its label should state that it has been so screened. There are no clear recommended dosages, but I think 1,000 to 4,000 mg a day is certainly very safe and effective.

The only people who need to be careful with taking omega-3 oils are people who are on pharmaceutical blood-thinning medications, and they should ask their doctor if they can take it, and at what dose.

Curcumin (Turmeric Root)

Very recent research has shown that *curcumin* is a very powerful anti-inflammatory and anti-oxidant substance, and is a potential therapeutic agent for arthritis, allergies, Alzheimer's, certain cancers, obesity, diabetes, and autoimmune diseases. Once again, we're seeing the direct correlation between inflammation and many of the cortisol-related diseases I mentioned in earlier chapters.

The standard dose is 650 mg three times a day, and curcumin works much better when taken with fat, such as the omega-3 oils, or a tablespoon of olive oil.

The only people who need to be careful with taking curcumin are those with a history of kidney stones and gall bladder stones.

Resveratrol

Resveratrol comes from the skins of grapes and other berries and is a very powerful *antioxidant.*, Antioxidants are a group of substances that help the body sweep out harmful molecules called free radicals. Resveratrol has also proved to be a very powerful anti-inflammatory agent, especially with regard to reducing cytokines. The standard dose for resveratrol is 200 mg three times a day.

Restoring Hormone Balance

Once the repair of the intestinal tract is under way, it's time to consider nutritional support for the adrenal glands.

Once again, it's impossible to overemphasize the importance of carrying out the intestinal tract repair first. By neglecting to do so, all other attempts to rebalance the adrenal glands are doomed to failure, because the adrenals will continue to produce cortisol until they finally burn out and go into the adrenal fatigue phase of hypofunction. This doesn't mean that every case of adrenal dysfunction has to be accompanied by intestinal tract inflammation, but it's always wise to check for it before proceeding with supplements for hormonal support.

This brings us to the topic of *glandular extracts*, which are nutritional supplements made from specific animal organs, usually bovine (cattle).

Glandular extracts were widely used by medical doctors at the beginning of the last century and were manufactured by pharmaceutical companies such as Eli Lilly and Upjohn as recently as the late 1960s. These days, many medical doctors have little regard for glandular extracts and consider them to be nothing more than "meat pills" (a matter that I will address shortly). This position ignores the medical history of glandular extracts.

During the 1919 flu pandemic, a certain Dr. Lucke at Camp Zachary Taylor (a military camp in Kentucky) found, upon autopsy, that 106 out of 126 individuals who died from the virus exhibited damaged adrenal glands. The damage was due to the sheer strain the illness placed on the victims' adrenals. Several hundred infected people treated with adrenal glandular extracts experienced less severe symptoms as well as dramatically reduced recovery periods.

With the advent in the 1950s of antibiotics and cortisone (synthetic cortisol, three times more powerful than the natural form), medications specifically developed to fight infection and inflammation, medical doctors simply turned away from glandular extracts and began prescribing mass quantities of these new wonder drugs. Unfortunately, by the time the significant negative side effects of cortisone became clear, medical doctors were sold on a drug that could only be obtained by prescription—and that generated windfall profits for the pharmaceutical company that manufactured it. And while there's no doubt that antibiotics have saved countless lives, the overuse of these drugs has now created the problem of drug-resistant bacteria, as well as promoting intestinal tract inflammation in a significant percentage of the population.

So what are we to make of glandular extracts? Once ingested, aren't they burned up by the stomach's hydrochloric acid? Even if they are absorbed intact, how do they affect the specific organs they're intended for? Aren't glandular extracts really nothing more than dried "meat pills"?

In the References section, I provide the information necessary for you to find the primary sources for all the dry scientific studies on glandular extracts, but what they boil down to is this: no, these are not simply dried "meat pills". Glandular extracts are not burned up by the stomach's hydrochloric acid; they are easily absorbed intact by the digestive tract; and they do go directly to the target tissue and support that tissue's function.

As an example, research proves that orally-ingested thymus glandular extract makes its way to the thymus gland and improves the production, maturation, and activation of immune system T-cells; and because glandular extracts can specifically reach the target tissue (e.g., adrenal, hypothalamus, pituitary), they are highly beneficial to the nutritional restoration of the corresponding gland. By correlating the results of the ASI test with the person's symptoms, a nutritional supplement program can be designed to meet the specific needs of each patient.

When the ASI shows that the cortisol level is too low in any phase of the test, particularly if the adrenal glands are in a state of fatigue, then supplementation with adrenal glandular extracts is appropriate in restoring adrenal health. The dosage will vary depending on how depleted the adrenal glands are as well as the quality of the glandular extract being used; a doctor who is well-versed in using these extracts will be your best resource.

For those patients who prefer not to use glandular products, Apex offers a herbal supplement called AdrenaStim in the form of an easy-to-use skin cream for adrenal fatigue.

The adrenal supplementation program does not always require glandular extracts (which are problematic for vegetarians); in fact, sometimes these are simply not appropriate in treating cortisol imbalances. Adrenal glandular extracts can elevate cortisol levels, so taking them obviously isn't going to resolve a cortisol imbalance where the cortisol is already too high.

In this case we would use a supplement called ADHS (Biotics) or Adaptocrine (Apex), which lowers or stabilizes cortisol levels. ADHS and Adaptocrine contain a balance of vitamins and Chinese and Ayurvedic herbs that nutritionally support normal cortisol and DHEA levels. Keeping in mind that the ASI test measures the cortisol levels four times throughout the day, the supplement program can easily be tailored to the specific fluctuations in cortisol levels.

Once again, if you don't have access to a doctor who offers these supplements, the alternative is to buy some ginseng, holy basil, and rhodiola at about 200 mg of each, and take these three times a day. These are considered *adaptogenic* (creating or promoting adaptation) herbs which will support normal cortisol levels throughout the day.

The point to remember is that cortisol imbalances have lots of twists and turns, and it isn't as simple as the cortisol just being either too low or too high. This is why the ASI test can be so helpful, because cortisol can be normal during one part of the day, too low during another part, and then too high at yet another. **This is the reason why it's important to treat each case on an individual basis** and not to assume that the supplement program that works for one patient is going to yield similar results for the next patient.

DHEA

DHEA is important in helping the adrenals maintain the proper cortisol/DHEA ratios, which will be part of the ASI test results. If the cortisol and DHEA levels are too low, then a DHEA supplement may be required.

Nobody should take DHEA if their cortisol levels are high because the body can convert DHEA to cortisol, as well as to testosterone, estrogen, and progesterone. This is why cortisol imbalances should be managed by a doctor experienced in this area, and why you shouldn't just run to the vitamin store every time you read an article that touts the next new fountain-of-youth supplement. If you're a woman who might be at risk for breast, uterine, or ovarian cancer, DHEA is definitely not a good idea.

Once again, the dosage of DHEA will vary depending on the results of the ASI, but most of the time a dose between 5 and 10 mg is all that is required.

Liver Repair and Detoxification

There are other supplements that are not only useful but necessary to fully repair all the damage caused by cortisol imbalances.

Sometimes the liver becomes overburdened from the continual return of toxins leaking through the intestinal wall, in which case nutrients that support detoxification are needed. Another possible factor in liver toxicity are *xenobiotics*, foreign agents that include plastics, organic solvents, pesticides, industrial wastes in water and air, and some medications.

Most of the supplements that assist in liver detoxification are antioxidants that eliminate or neutralize free radicals. The appropriate nutritional supplements for liver detoxification are: milk thistle, curcumin, and a good quality multiple vitamin supplement.

It's important to note that the liver is also responsible for activating some hormones, such as thyroid and estrogen, and also has to break down excess hormones. If the liver isn't working properly, it may be just another trigger for a host of hormone imbalances.

Fixing the Thermostat

There's absolutely no point in taking the nutritional supplements I've recommended if we don't also make sure that the hypothalamus and pituitary gland are working okay.

This is a point I repeatedly bring up when I teach this material to doctors: just as you can't fix any of this unless you repair the intestinal tract, you also can't fix the problems we're discussing if the structures that control all hormonal activity aren't working.

All that's needed here is a hypothalamus/pituitary gland supplement. The Biotics product is Cytozyme PT/HPT, and the Apex one is called MasterZyme, but you can usually find a supplement like this at a very good vitamin store. The glandular extracts used come from lamb rather than cows so as to avoid any possibility of, or questions about, Mad Cow disease (BSE).

To address this need on your own, you would buy *phosphatidylserine* at a vitamin store and take 100 mg three times a day.

The Importance of L-tyrosine in Adrenal and Thyroid Hormone Production

The last nutritional supplement that can play a significant role in resolving cortisol imbalances is the amino acid L-tyrosine, which also can have a beneficial effect on thyroid and brain function. In order for the adrenal glands and the thyroid gland to produce hormones, L-tyrosine must be adequately absorbed in the intestinal tract from protein. As well as helping to regulate body temperature, L-tyrosine is also used by the nervous system to make dopamine, which relays nerve transmissions.

In my clinical experience, L-tyrosine can be enormously useful in (i) patients who are in adrenal fatigue; (ii) those whose hands and feet (if not their whole bodies) are cold most of the time; and (iii), those who are easily depressed.

I've seen the best results in cases that involve women with a family history of thyroid problems and who often show only low-normal or even normal results on a thyroid blood test, even though they have the classic hypothyroid symptoms of fatigue, coldness, and depression. In these cases there may be a genetic inability to absorb tyrosine from the proteins in the diet; but when these patients take a tyrosine supplement on an empty stomach (no protein present), they can absorb it quite well. Often the patient shows an improvement in all their symptoms after just a week of tyrosine supplementation (500 mg twice a day on an empty stomach to ensure complete absorption).

L-tyrosine, however, is absolutely not for everybody, and it must be used **carefully**. L-tyrosine can raise blood pressure and should never be used in people who have hypertension, even if they have hypothyroid symptoms. For the same reason, L-tyrosine should not be used by those who are prone to vascular headaches or migraine headaches. Lastly, L-tyrosine should never be taken in conjunction with antidepressant drugs containing monoamine oxidase (MAO) inhibitors, as the blood pressure could rise to very high levels.

Chromium

Chromium is a trace mineral that has been found to be very effective in controlling sugar cravings since it affects insulin regulation. It can also be useful in lowering cholesterol levels, especially triglycerides, as elevated cholesterol is more a problem of carbohydrate management than fat consumption. Chromium is important in cases of insulin resistance and diabetes.

The most effective dosages I have found are 200 mcg twice a day. If craving sugar is part of your hormonal symptoms, you absolutely need to add this to your 3R Program. Chromium can be easily bought in a vitamin store, and is one supplement that is very safe and that probably everyone should be taking.

A Review of the 3R Program

(Note: because of its key importance, this is also reprinted in the appendix as a handy reference)

Repair the intestinal tract:

- L-glutamine: 1,500 mg morning and night on an empty stomach for six to eight weeks; if good progress is made, you can drop to 1,500 mg just once a day as preventative maintenance thereafter.

- Psyllium or guar gum fiber at roughly 6 to 10 grams morning and night in either capsule or powdered form as directed on the supplement's label.

- Probiotics: as recommended on label.

- Curcumin: 650 mg two times a day (already a part of the Resolve aspect of the program, below) with food.

- Resveratrol: 200 mg three times a day with food.

- Optional: acetyl-l carnitine 500 mg and alpha lipoic acid 250 mg (for good glutathione levels), once a day with food.

- After 6-8 weeks of taking L-glutamine: begin oregano oil as directed on label with food if a Candida yeast problem exists.

NO WONDER YOU FEEL LIKE CRAP!

Resolve inflammation:

- Omega-3 oils: 2,000 mg two times a day with food.

- Curcumin: 650 mg two times a day (which you're already taking in the Repair aspect of the program, above).

Restore hormone balance:

This can only be addressed accurately with an ASI or other hormone test. If you're not working with a doctor who can give you the specific Biotics or Apex supplements I use, you may safely try the following:

- Chromium: 200 mcg twice a day for blood sugar support with food.

- Ginseng, holy basil, rhodiola: 200 mg of each three times a day with food for adrenal gland support.

- Phosphatidylserine: 100 mg three times a day with food for pituitary/hypothalamus support.

- Vitamin D3: 2,000 IU a day with food.

- Multiple vitamin and mineral supplement: for a really good quality one, go to a vitamin store, as this will ensure that you will get the B vitamins, vitamin C, and the minerals your body needs to function properly. You can't always assume that you're getting everything you need out of the foods you're eating even with a good diet. Check the label to see how much chromium the supplement contains; if it has 200mcg or more, then you won't have to take extra chromium (indicated in the Repair aspect of the program, above).

The Maintenance 3R Program

Once you have regained your health you're going to want to keep it that way and not let yourself gradually relapse and have to start all over again.

As I mentioned in the preface of this book, we live in challenging times, besieged by environmental toxins, genetically modified foods, and a virtual sea of estrogen from all the plastics that surround us. In order to remain healthy, your best bet is to stay on a maintenance 3R Program, as follows

- L-glutamine: 1,500 mg once a day on an empty stomach.

- Curcumin: 650 mg once a day.

- Psyllium or guar gum fiber at roughly 6 to 10 grams morning and night in either capsule or powdered form as directed on the supplement's label.

- Resveratrol: 200 mg once a day.

- Vitamin D3: 1,000 mg once a day.

- Omega-3 oil: 1,000 mg morning and night.

- Multiple vitamin: as directed on label.

MAKE THE PAIN GO AWAY

Treating Causes instead of Symptoms

Chronic pain usually results in long-term use of NSAIDs (nonsteriodal anti-inflammatory medications such as aspirin and ibuprofen) which, as we have seen, eventually leads to intestinal tract inflammation and leaky gut syndrome, which in turn leads to cortisol imbalances and a host of other problems. It's obviously important to try to resolve the cause(s) of the pain rather than continue to merely treat the symptoms.

Referring back to the components of the triangle of health, if a structural component (e.g., knee, vertebra, elbow) is compromised, thereby causing pain and stress to the body, then the pain must be resolved in order to keep cortisol levels balanced.

Over the years, there's been so much misinformation regarding the cause of and appropriate treatment for joint pain—whether back, neck, or other joints—that it has become very difficult for patients to decide what type of therapy is best for their condition. Fortunately, following years of extensive research, there's now a compelling amount of evidence supporting the positive effects of spinal and joint manipulation. One of the most comprehensive research studies comes from the U.S. Department of Health and its Agency for Health Care Policy and Research (AHCPR), which was established to determine what are the most effective forms of treatment for specific disorders.

In December 1994, this multidisciplinary panel recommended spinal manipulation as a highly effective treatment for lower back pain. Another research study done at Duke University in 2000 proved that spinal manipulation is very effective for treating headaches and ranked it as a superior form of treatment when compared to prescription drugs, over-the-counter drugs, and acupuncture. These studies did not specifically use the term chiropractic, but the reality is that with the exception of some osteopaths, chiropractors are the only doctors specifically trained and qualified to perform spinal and joint manipulation.

Chiropractic care has several different adjusting techniques for performing spinal manipulation, most of which are extremely gentle. The perception that chiropractic adjustments resemble something out of World Federation Wrestling is grossly erroneous. There are methods of spinal manipulation or adjustment that use a handheld instrument which delivers a precisely measured thrust to the joint; other times a gentle thrust of the thumb is all that is needed. Sometimes simply having the patient lie on strategically placed cushioned wedges that adjust the pelvic girdle is all that is required. These methods are also ideal for adjusting other joints, such as shoulders, knees, and elbows. The Resource Guide at the end of this book will help direct you to doctors who perform these techniques.

Where the Pain is Coming From

Since its inception in 1895, chiropractic philosophy has embraced the concept that the nerves exiting the spinal cord between the vertebrae control most of the body's functions, and that the ability of these spinal nerves to properly transmit messages between the brain and the rest of the body can become altered or compromised if there is a dysfunction in vertebral joint mechanics. The belief was that if the spinal nerves were being pinched or compressed, this would alter their ability to function normally.

While this phenomenon does occur and does cause pain, which is more likely to radiate down an arm or a leg than to be felt locally, it's not the sole reason for joint pain.

Fortunately, through recent advances in neuroscience, we now know that the primary basis for joint pain involves the nerve cells **inside** the joints. These cells, called *mechanoreceptors*, are concerned with the mechanical function of the joint as well as with *proprioception*, or balance.

In numerous studies involving automobile whiplash injuries, researchers have concluded that the damage that causes pain has struck either the spinal joints and/or the discs between the vertebrae; and we know that both of these structures are loaded with mechanoreceptor nerve cells. In this type of injury, the joint's ability to move in its normal functional range has been compromised by traumatic impact, which results in the understimulation of the mechanoreceptors—essentially, the joint is stuck in a position that doesn't allow for adequate mechanoreceptor stimulation. This is also the case in lifting injuries, sports injuries, and even cases of sleeping in the wrong position.

If enough of the mechanoreceptors in any given joint are sufficiently understimulated, it activates or turns on the mechanoreceptor pain fibers, which fire pain stimuli to the brain. Damage to the discs also results in poor mechanoreceptor innervations (nerve supply), and in pain. This is a major reason most people with spinal or other types of joint pain find that they are often in more pain in the morning after they have been lying still for six to eight hours and improve somewhat after moving around—in effect, having their mechanoreceptors restimulated.

Another interesting facet of this is how so many people with joint pain swear they feel better after a hot morning shower, which leads them to believe that heat is beneficial to their condition. The reality is that the only other place in the human body that has mechanoreceptor nerve cells is the skin. What is actually happening is that the water from the shower head is stimulating the skin and the mechanoreceptors, and any time you stimulate the mechanoreceptors, the pain will abate.

The reason manipulation of spinal and other joints (as performed by chiropractors and osteopaths) relieves pain is that it restores the joint to its normal range of motion and enables the mechanoreceptors to regain normal stimulation, effectively treating the cause, not just the symptom.

Recent research with advanced imaging techniques that can track a marker for inflammation now tells us that **all pain has an inflammatory component**; this inflammation, sadly, can continue even after the injured tissue has healed. Inflammation can also increase the perception of pain, which helps to explain chronic pain syndromes. This again illustrates the need to reduce the inflammatory response by using the 3R Program.

How it's All Wired Together

There's an enormous neurological consequence to mechanoreceptor dysfunction which is related to how these cells are wired into the spinal cord.

Mechanoreceptors synapse or fire into a place called the seventh *lamina* (layer) of the spinal cord, which is also where we find the nerve fibers that go to muscles, the immune system, the vascular system, the adrenal glands, and most other organs. Therefore, chiropractors also believe that many health disorders, including those involving organ function, may have their basis in mechanoreceptor dysfunction that can benefit from spinal manipulation, which chiropractors also call spinal *adjustments.*

An example of the far-reaching neurological effects of spinal manipulation can be found in a current research study that shows that spinal manipulation directly decreases cortisol secretion and, therefore, dramatically increases immune function. This is an ongoing study from Australia into the effects of spinal manipulation on asthma, depression, and anxiety. The study began in 2002 and involves 420 patients with an average age of forty-six. Other forms of manual therapy, such as massage, were also tested, but researchers found that only the group that received spinal manipulation displayed significant improvement in asthma symptoms, depression, and anxiety scores.

Chiropractic care takes into account the triangle of health and addresses its structural, chemical, and emotional components. Chiropractic care can include: spinal and other joint manipulation; physiotherapy modalities such as ultrasound; nutritional counseling; hormone testing and balancing programs; postural education; strengthening and stretching programs; and techniques for neuro-emotional stability.

If you've been suffering from a pain syndrome that simply will not resolve with medical care, or if the symptoms are only alleviated by taking medication that sooner or later is going to produce an unwanted side effect, then you're an excellent candidate for chiropractic care. The ultimate goal of chiropractic care is to treat the **cause** as opposed to the **symptom;** and since the nervous system is connected to nearly every one of your cells, it's not hard to understand that neurological imbalances can have far-reaching health consequences. If you don't find a way to resolve your pain, and the stress it inflicts on your body, it's hard to imagine how you will keep your cortisol levels balanced.

In the event you've tried everything from traditional medical care, chiropractic care, acupuncture, physical therapy, all the way to witch doctors and still can't find relief, there are three factors that have probably been overlooked. These three factors are: psoas muscle spasm, ligament instability, and a craniosacral syndrome.

The Importance of Psoas Muscle Balance

One of the first things that can go wrong when a lower back, hip joint, shoulder, or neck problem won't resolve is that there is probably an undetected psoas muscle spasm.

The psoas muscles are two of the most important muscles in the lower back, one on each side. They attach the ball of the hip to the socket of the pelvis; they are firmly attached to the front of all five of the lower back vertebrae, including the discs; and they end at the last two vertebrae that have ribs attached to them (technically, the bottom of the shoulder girdle).

The psoas muscles are responsible for two functions. When they contract individually, they cause the knee to flex toward the waist as in walking, running, climbing stairs, or riding a bicycle. When both psoas muscles contract at the same time, you're either lying on your back pulling your knees up toward your chest or you're bending over at the waist—and bending over at the waist is what gets most people into trouble with their lower backs. Since lower back pain is a leading cause of people seeing a doctor, each day doctor's offices around the world are filled with patients who tell a tale of woe about how they injured their backs by lifting while bending or simply by reaching forward. In many cases they weren't even lifting something heavy, and the movement could have been as innocuous as putting on their socks.

What's happened is that their psoas muscles are already overly tight, and as they engage in forward bending activities, it becomes a case of the straw that breaks the camel's back: It's just one time too many. At that point they are so close to the muscle going into a full-scale spasm that it only takes a few more forward movements for the spasm to occur. Sometimes it can go into spasm as the end result of repetitive flexion activities, such as gardening or house cleaning.

When this occurs, patients often describe feeling as though their back "went out" or "gave way." What they're describing is the dramatic effect of one of the psoas muscles becoming so spastic that it pulls the lumbar spine and pelvic girdle into a fixated position that no longer enables it to function within its normal range of motion. As previously discussed, this results in the understimulation of the mechanoreceptor nerves and triggers the pain fibers. The pain can range from discomfort to complete debilitation, preventing the patient from standing up straight or walking properly.

People with chronic lower back pain will frequently notice that the pain can travel upward and result in neck or shoulder pain. It's always interesting when, during a consultation with a new patient, they first tell me all about their history of lower back pain and then at some later point they mention a shoulder problem they have acquired without incurring any injury or trauma. It never occurs to them that the two problems are related.

Because the psoas muscles are attached to the bottom of the shoulder girdle, when one muscle goes into spasm, it pulls down on the shoulder to create an anatomical and physiological imbalance. It's hard to predict which shoulder will have pain, as it could be the one that's too low or the one that's too high. Similarly, it's just as difficult to predict which side of the lower back might be more painful relative to which psoas muscle has gone into spasm, and it's not unusual for the pain to be worse on the side opposite the muscle spasm.

Most certainly, not everyone with lower back, hip, shoulder, or neck pain has a psoas muscle involvement, but if you're the unlucky person who tends to incur this muscle imbalance, you're not going to achieve a level of continued stability if it's not corrected. Instead, you will be the person who fears the next episode of lower back pain that you're sure is coming from some simple activity that requires bending over from the waist. The truly good news is that it takes exactly ten seconds to correct it, and you can do it lying in bed at home. In my next book I'm going to tell you how.

Oh, okay, then—we'll take care of this now.

The technique for correcting a psoas muscle spasm is so easy that most patients try to mess it up and make it more complicated than necessary. Since we can't be sure which muscle is involved without properly examining you, the next best thing is to do the corrective procedure on both sides, which is completely safe. The technique is identical for both sides, so while the instructions I'm giving are for a right psoas muscle spasm, obviously you would just reverse it to resolve the left psoas muscle.

1. Lie on your back in bed and bend your right knee up, keeping your right foot flat on the bed

2. Place your left hand one inch to the right of your navel.

3. Press your left hand gently down into your abdomen and, while holding that pressure, slowly swing your right knee toward your left leg ten times, still keeping your right foot flat on the bed. This will feel like you're doing absolutely nothing of any benefit because most of the time it causes no pain or discomfort. If you're thinking nothing is happening, you're mistaken. I promise you that this simple procedure will resolve the psoas spasm.

4. Repeat this procedure on the left side.

There's a logic I impart to my patients when I teach them to do the psoas correction, which is that while it's very important that they get back into proper alignment, it's equally important that they **stay** that way. If I put a patient back in alignment and neglect to correct a psoas muscle spasm, just how long should we expect that patient to stay in alignment considering that he or she is going to have to use his psoas muscle to walk out of my office? It's my guess the patient will be lucky to make it to their car before the spastic psoas muscle begins to pull them off-center again.

These are the kinds of patients who will say they have trouble "holding" their adjustments, or they give up treatment because they don't stay well for very long. Or if it isn't their lower back that hurts then it's their neck, or their shoulders, or it's always something. They never achieve meaningful stability, and they also develop a well-deserved paranoia about their bodies because they feel they are walking time bombs; every time they bend forward or reach for something, they might suddenly end up in pain. They grow wary of activities that used to be fun for fear of hurting themselves, and it limits their quality of life.

If you happen to be one of these unlucky souls, then your best defense is to do the psoas muscle corrective procedure every morning before you get out of bed and every night when you get back into bed. You can also do it before and after an activity that will require some flexion, such as gardening. It's important to understand that you're trying to prevent a problem from occurring, so you should do this even if you're not experiencing pain—just as you brush your teeth every day, not just when they hurt.

Since the psoas muscles are responsible for the ability to bend from the waist, and that activity causes more lower back pain than anything else, it's equally important that you learn to **bend your knees** to reach for things that are lower than you are. It's not just when lifting heavy objects that it's important to bend your knees, beause it's the repetitive strain on the psoas muscles that gets a lot of us into trouble.

It takes human beings about thirty days to develop a new muscle memory pattern, and considering you've been bending over incorrectly for most of your life, you have to be patient with yourself in learning to bend with your knees. No doubt, after two weeks you will still catch yourself bending incorrectly, but if you persevere for the whole thirty days, you will get the hang of it. Ideally, you want to reach a point where you almost never bend over at the waist, and if you have to, you're **still** bending your knees to transfer the strain from your lower back to your thigh muscles.

If your spinal or other joints are fixated and not in normal alignment, however, doing the psoas corrective procedure alone will not put you back in alignment. You will still need to see a chiropractor or an osteopath who does manipulation if you're ever going to recover. The point is, if you're out of alignment and that's the cause of your pain or symptoms, you're not going to get better until you get back into alignment. You can put ice on it, use heat, do ultrasound, rub it, medicate it, and even perform surgery on it, but in the end you're still out of alignment and in a state of neurological dysfunction.

By no means should this be construed to mean that chiropractic or manipulative care is appropriate for every condition: I can assure you that if you ever saw me carve a Thanksgiving turkey, you would **not** want me performing your appendectomy! Manipulative care is obviously not the treatment of choice for broken bones, cancers, or pathological or psychiatric diseases.

Achieving Ligament Stability

The second problem I most frequently notice when a person in pain has tried chiropractic or manipulative care and either hasn't fully recovered or achieved lasting stability, is that he or she hasn't been properly instructed on the importance of cold compress therapy.

Nearly everything that goes wrong with joints, ligaments, tendons, and muscles involves inflammation. From a medical perspective, this is why anti-inflammatory medications are prescribed. One of the major problems with this approach, aside from the intestinal tract inflammation side effects described earlier, is that these medications don't work very well with respect to joint and ligament injuries. Joints and ligaments are by and large *avascular*, which means they have a minimal blood supply. This makes it hard for a medication taken orally and delivered through the bloodstream to effectively reach these tissues.

As a chiropractor, I often reflect on the fact that if anti-inflammatory medications worked as well on joint and ligament problems as medical doctors and patients hoped, there wouldn't be so much need for chiropractic care. Instead, the single most common phenomenon in any chiropractic office is the new patient who has a history of using NSAIDs and is complaining about how the NSAIDs didn't relieve his or her pain.

Although the use of cold compresses is often recommended, especially in the acute phase of an injury or pain syndrome, the patient is usually not instructed properly as to how long to use them, or even given the rationale for their use. When I see patients who have been told to use cold compresses but still don't get well, the reason is always the same: they were told to use the cold compresses only at the onset of pain and to use them only for the first three days. This is both incredibly shortsighted and guarantees failure.

First, the inflammation is definitely going to last more than three days. I find it very interesting that the same doctor who tells patients to use cold compresses for only three days will, at the same time, put them on a **one-month** prescription of NSAIDs. The application of cold compresses to resolve inflammation **must** be used on a consistent, long-term basis, often for as long as four to six weeks.

Second, and most important, ligaments—the tissues that hold the joints together—are also the slowest-healing tissue in the body. If the ligaments don't fully heal and regain the tensile strength necessary to hold the joints in proper functional alignment, then a complete recovery may never occur, increasing the chance of reinjury. In this situation, the patient finds that every time they engage in strenuous activity they run the risk of recurring pain because they're placing stress on ligaments that have never fully healed and are therefore unable to keep the joints stable. If you combine this problem of ligament instability with an undetected psoas-muscle spasm, it's easy to see how much trouble a person can get into with activities requiring bending forward. It's a generally accepted fact that ligaments take a minimum of four to six weeks to repair, although there is research that states it could take longer, depending on the degree of trauma involved.

Ligaments are composed primarily of collagen, whose molecules bind together in a cold environment, just like the gelatin product, Jell-O. While Jell-O has to be heated up on the stove to get all the ingredients to combine evenly, it won't acquire that wobbly, gelatinous consistency until it's placed in the refrigerator. Jell-O contains much less collagen than your ligaments do, which is a good thing, unless you want to be Gumby or a contortionist. By using cold compresses on a joint or ligament injury for the entire four to six weeks required to heal the ligaments, you're giving them the opportunity to fully bind together and regain their normal tensile strength.

Another reason for using cold compresses on areas where ligaments are subjected to stress is the prevention of injuries. My favorite story about this subject involves a forty-two-year-old male in the concrete-pouring business who came to see me with a history of chronic lower back pain. He went through a typical course of treatment, became completely pain-free, and was released from further treatment. My parting advice to him was that if he wanted to reduce the risk of another injury, he should use cold compresses on his lower back every day that he worked in order to prevent the ligaments from becoming progressively weakened.

I have given this advice over and over again for many years and frankly, hardly anyone listens! The reason for this is the brain's ability to forget pain—and without the pain to remind us, we simply stop doing the things that would prevent it.

About two and a half years later, this patient returned to my office for care. Being a creature of presumption, I asked what was wrong with his lower back. He surprised me by saying that his lower back was fine, but he had slept on his stomach and woken up with neck pain. My curiosity regarding his lower back was no less diminished, and I asked him about it again since it had been such a long time between visits. He told me that he had actually used the cold compresses on his back every day after work, and the pain had never returned.

The point here is that the use of cold compresses can be preventative as well as curative. Unfortunately, most of us have been raised by mothers who dragged out the heating pad for every ache and pain, and we have a measure of doubt about using cold because it sounds like it may be uncomfortable. In reality, the cold is very soothing and brings an almost immediate sense of relief. However, for it to be effective, it must be used properly and sensibly.

First of all, we're talking about cold compresses and not the **direct** application of ice to the skin. This can best be accomplished by using a soft gel pack, which can be found in most pharmacies, and putting it in the freezer until it gets cold. The trick of turning an ice pack into a cold pack involves nothing more than placing a towel between the pack and your skin. As people have different tolerances to cold, I advise my patients to put enough towels and/or clothing in between so that they are comfortable. The sensation you should feel while using the cold compress should cause a sigh of relief, an "Ah, that feels good" experience.

The cold compress should be applied for twenty minutes at a time and no longer. It's not a case of the longer you use it, the better the result. However, it's true that the more **frequently** you use the cold compresses, the faster you will heal. For the average working person with the typically busy schedule, the best one can hope for is using the compresses twice a day: perhaps once before or after dinner and then again before bedtime. On days off or on weekends, the frequency of application could be increased. You should allow one hour between applications.

When Heat can Help

There's a place for therapies that use heat, but most of the time it involves the types that will be found in either a doctor's or a physical therapist's office. Therapies such as ultrasound or short-wave diathermy have value because of their ability to penetrate from one to four inches into the body and alter the chemistry of the muscles. The old heating pad at home has very poor penetration capabilities and will not have much effect on the lactic acid content of a spastic muscle. The primary value in using heat therapies on tight muscles is to remove lactic acid that can become congested in the muscle.

Muscles use glucose for fuel and give off lactic acid as a waste product of this process. Under normal circumstances, once the muscle relaxes, the lactic acid gets dumped out into the circulatory system, where it's transported to the kidneys and excreted into the urine. However, if the muscles remain in a state of abnormal prolonged contraction due to an aberrant nerve supply, the lactic acid will become trapped inside and cause further problems.

Let's take an example. The patient is out of alignment, so the nerves going to a particular muscle group are overly excited and are causing the muscles to go into spasm. Unlike physical exercise, in which the muscles relax once that activity ceases, the muscles getting the excessive nerve signals remain contracted (keep in mind that muscles only do what the nerves tell them to do). The only exception to this is the presence of some other chemical imbalance in the muscle, such as a calcium deficiency, which is rare, or a disease like Parkinson's).

So now the chiropractor is trying to get the patient back into alignment, but the tight muscles are resisting and pulling the alignment out again.

Although there's plenty of research to prove that spinal manipulation will cause muscles to relax, sometimes the muscle is so badly congested with lactic acid that it rebounds and goes back into spasm. The problem is that if the concentration of lactic acid inside the muscle becomes too high, it'll cause the muscle to contract further. The muscle becomes stuck in a cycle of abnormal nerve supply, causing a spasm and a buildup of lactic acid, which just perpetuates the condition.

An excess of lactic acid is responsible for the burning type of pain people experience in their muscles. In the early days of aerobic dance classes, it was popular for the instructors to urge participants to "feel the burn." This fell out of fashion as it became apparent that the muscles were actually being overused and damaged.

Research on Olympic athletes shows that cold compresses disperse lactic acid from muscles as well as heat does; but in the case of prolonged spasms, there again is the problem of effectively penetrating the muscle. This is where ultrasound or short-wave diathermy can be useful, since these techniques use sound or radio waves to push the heat deep into the muscle tissue, thereby dispersing the lactic acid. By clearing the lactic acid out, the muscle has a better chance of resuming its relaxed state while the nervous system is being normalized by spinal manipulation.

It's also worth mentioning that drinking sufficient amounts of water is essential to the body's elimination of lactic acid. If you find you get stiff muscles easily with activity or exercise, then you're probably not drinking enough water, and you could be putting yourself at risk of injury due to overly tight muscles.

To conclude this brief discourse on heat therapies, cold compresses at home are still the best way to go for most pain syndromes, whether they are acute or chronic. As I stated earlier, the failure to use cold compresses properly constitutes the second factor in the list of problems that can prevent recovery from joint and ligament injuries.

Craniosacral Therapy

The third factor that might account for a patient's failure to recover is that there is something wrong with their head, literally and structurally. Fortunately, in both the chiropractic and osteopathic arsenals there's a treatment known as *craniosacral therapy*.

The premise of craniosacral therapy deals with an aspect of human physiology known as the *primary respiratory mechanism*, which refers to the movement of *cerebrospinal fluid* from the brain down through the spinal cord. One of the most important features of craniosacral function is that a rhythmic motion occurs at the sutures where the bones of the skull meet and that there is a corresponding motion in the membranes covering the brain and the spinal cord.

The *sacral* part refers to the last bony segment of the spinal column that people commonly call their tailbone, which also has a rhythmic motion that is synchronized with the cranial bones. Because the cerebrospinal fluid is the medium that transports all the oxygen and nutrients used by the brain and the spinal nerves, the ability of the cranial bones to move normally and assist in the flow of this fluid is vitally important.

The traditional medical community initially rejected this concept of cranial motion because—according to accepted curricula—the sutures of the skull become fused by the age of twenty-five. The idea that these bones could move and, even worse, become misaligned and thereby adversely affect human health was met with great derision.

One of the first doctors to advance the concept of craniosacral motion was an osteopath named William Sutherland. In 1939, to prove that the sutures did not fuse together, he performed an experiment whose simplicity and brilliance you just have to love.

Dr. Sutherland took the skull of a fresh cadaver, cleaned it out until all the tissue was gone, and filled the inside of the skull with dried beans. He then placed the skull in a large pot of water and went to bed. Upon arising the next morning he found that the sutures of the skull had disarticulated and separated because of the expansion of the beans.

Of course, the medical community thought Dr. Sutherland was the one full of beans, and craniosacral motion remained a controversial subject. In the end, Dr. Sutherland had the last laugh (albeit from the confines of his grave) when researchers at Michigan State University College of Osteopathic Medicine confirmed cranial motion using X-ray studies of living skulls.

Craniosacral therapy has been around a long time in both the chiropractic and osteopathic professions, although not all chiropractors and even fewer osteopaths practice it. Many chiropractors use, among other approaches, an adjusting method called *sacral occipital technique*. Within the osteopathic profession there has been a resurgence of interest in craniosacral therapy largely in response to the efforts of Dr. John E. Upledger. The Upledger Institute teaches a comprehensive series of craniosacral classes, and although I'm not sure how many osteopaths are learning this technique, I can guarantee that legions of physical and massage therapists are.

The cranial bones can become misaligned in a variety of ways, including the very process of being born. In the days before natural birth became popular, many doctors refused to believe that a baby could navigate its way through the birth canal without the help of forceps. Needless to say, grabbing the soft skull of an infant with a large pair of pliers and pulling on it is an excellent way to bestow a cranial misalignment. Even today, although forceps are used much less frequently, there is still the cranial suction cap that pulls on the infant's skull.

Should you manage to survive your birth with your cranial alignment intact, there are always the misadventures of childhood and the inevitable injuries and accidents of everyday life which can cause cranial problems. Anyone who's witnessed an infant trying to learn to walk can easily understand how the cranium can become misaligned as the struggling infant spends more time falling down than standing up. During childhood a host of possible head injuries can occur, ranging from innocent falls and sports injuries to (sadly) outright child abuse.

If the craniosacral function is unbalanced, it will translate to spinal imbalance. The cervical spine (*aka* the neck) which the skull is sitting on, as well as the lower back/sacral area, will be directly affected; and as the mid-back tries to compensate for the imbalances occurring above and below, it too will have trouble staying properly aligned. It's usually quite easy for me to tell whether new patients have a craniosacral problem because they have nearly every box checked off on my symptom questionnaire!

This brings us back again to that elusive concept of stability. If craniosacral function is compromised, patients won't be able to stay in alignment no matter how many times they're treated by their chiropractor. If it turns out that your chiropractor isn't skilled in craniosacral therapy, then you simply need to find a physical or massage therapist who is, and let him or her resolve the imbalance in conjunction with having the chiropractor work on your spinal alignment.

Craniosacral therapy has now gained wide acceptance within the medical community, as they refer their patients with neck and back problems to physical therapists who are trained in it. However, if a patient is receiving craniosacral therapy but other parts of the spine are out of alignment, the patient is still going to have to see a chiropractor to gain stability, because physical therapists are neither trained nor licensed to perform this manipulation.

From a chiropractic perspective, if your alignment has been correctly evaluated and treated, the psoas muscle and craniosacral components addressed, and you've been given the proper home-care instructions regarding cold compresses, posture, corrective exercises, and stretches, then the structural component of your pain syndrome should be well on the road to recovery. But the chemical and emotional parts of the health triangle may still need to be considered, and we'll be covering them in the following chapters.

Unfortunately, in the real world, it doesn't always work like this. As stated previously, not every physical disorder is not going to respond to chiropractic care, which is why God created orthopedic specialists, acupuncturists, physical therapists, and neurosurgeons. Unless your pain obviously requires surgery, trying chiropractic care first is a safe and conservative approach to getting well; there are times, however, when it just doesn't get the job done, and what I try to impress upon my patients is that I don't care **how** they get well, just that they do get well. If I can't make it happen through chiropractic, then it's my responsibility to review other options with them.

Natural Pain Relief: Proteolytic Enzymes

These are enzymes that cause a chemical chain reaction in the body to break down proteins.

One of the very best proteolytic enzymes is *bromelain*, which is a naturally occurring enzyme found in pineapples. Research has shown that bromelain reduces *bradykinin* production, thus lowering its ability to irritate the pain fibers in joints. The most powerful of the pro-inflammatory irritants, bradykinin can cause pain and swelling, activate other pain-producing prostaglandins, and promote fibrous scar tissue; so being able to reduce it with bromelain is truly significant.

Other proteolytic enzymes that reduce inflammation and pain are *papain* and *pancreatin*. Most vitamin stores sell bromelain either separately or in combination with these other enzymes, and I believe that taking them all together achieves the best results. These proteolytic enzymes must be taken on an empty stomach, or they will just assist with the digestion of your food and not reach the inflammation sites. These supplements have no known negative side effects, so you can take rather large amounts.

Different manufacturers may vary the amount of each proteolytic enzyme contained in each pill, but on average there'll be 50 mg of bromelain, 50 mg of papain, and 50 mg of pancreatin. Initially I would recommend five pills five times a day, and after two weeks I suggest reducing the dosage to three pills three times a day until the condition is resolved.

There are also other supplements to consider in treating the pro-inflammatory state, such as ginger, turmeric, and antioxidants.

Ginger is a wonderful anti-inflammatory agent because it has the dual properties of reducing the prostaglandins that cause inflammation while at the same time protecting the lining of the stomach (you'll recall that the whole problem with NSAIDs is that they irritate the gastrointestinal lining and can cause the leaky gut/elevated-cortisol syndrome). Ginger can be as effective as NSAIDs in relieving joint swelling and stiffness, but it will not damage the intestinal lining and, in fact, will protect it.

Ginger can be consumed in many ways, ranging from the fresh root used to season foods, to teas, to capsules of dried ginger powder. The capsules are the most potent form of ginger and realistically the easiest way to consistently get it into your system. An effective dosage would be 1,000 mg taken four times a day with food.

Curcumin, a very powerful anti-inflammatory herb extracted from turmeric, has been shown in research studies to be as effective as cortisone and ibuprofen. Curcumin is a very important part of the 3R Program. An appropriate amount would be 650 mg three times a day with food.

Acupuncture

As everyone knows, acupuncture has been around for thousands of years and has been used successfully to treat all kinds of ailments in Asian societies. This is another mode of therapy that practitioners of Western medicine don't like because they can't figure out how it works and they aren't trained to perform it. As a result, they disclaim its effectiveness in treating a wide variety of illnesses based on the ever-popular mantra of "where's the research to support it?" (Fortunately, physicists and engineers show more intelligence. Although many aspects of quantum mechanical theory are poorly understood, much of the modern world is built on applications based on it: without quantum mechanics, we wouldn't have semiconductors, lasers, computers, digital cameras, and much more. One can benefit from a thing without fully understanding it.)

Although much about how acupuncture affects the way the body functions may not be understood, when it comes to suppressing pain, the research is compelling. Acupuncture has the ability to stimulate the release of opiate-like compounds in the brain, thereby blocking the perception of pain. While some Western practitioners insist this is a placebo effect, the fact that Chinese veterinarians use acupuncture as anesthesia when performing surgery on animals disproves it. Furthermore, when synthetic drugs that block the effects of opiates on brain cells are administered, the effects of acupuncture in relieving pain are lost.

So if your pain syndrome isn't responding well to chiropractic care, acupuncture can be an excellent option. This is not to say that the two are incompatible; in fact, for very chronic, stubborn problems pursuing acupuncture and chiropractic at the same time can be very beneficial.

Physical Therapy

Another very good approach to relieving pain syndromes may be physical therapy. Sometimes pain is so chronic that patients simply become deconditioned, which is a polite way of saying they get out of shape. If you've been in pain for a long time, it's likely that you have not been able to exercise and the ensuing, progressive muscle weakness may be putting too much stress on your ligaments and joints.

It's also possible that you're suffering from a muscle imbalance, whereby muscles that are supposed to complement and counterbalance each other can't do so because one of them has either become too weak or too strong relative to the other. An example of this problem, which doesn't even involve an injury or pain syndrome, is that of bodybuilders who lift weights unevenly. Without proper training and guidance, some bodybuilders seek to bulk up their "front" muscles. They want strong biceps in their arms and pectorals in their chests, but they neglect to strengthen the opposing muscles because these are less visible (at least to them). This is called front-loading, and it leads to joint dysfunction because of the unevenness in strength and disproportionate pulling on the joints.

Physical therapy is also essential in providing rehabilitation of a joint following surgery, such as knee or hip replacement, to make sure the strength and range of motion return to normal.

Physical therapy can also address problems associated with scar tissue. When any connective tissue in the body—whether ligament, tendon, muscle, or even skin—has been damaged, it will be repaired with scar tissue. The problem with scar tissue is that it's tougher and less flexible than the original tissue it's repairing and it has more pain-transmitting fibers. So although the tougher-tissue repair sounds like a good idea, it's not.

Let's say you have a joint whose normal range of motion is ninety degrees, but because of either a serious injury or a series of repetitive injuries, there's a fair amount of what is called scar-tissue infiltration. So now you want to move this joint ninety degrees, but the tougher scar tissue embedded along with the normal tissue will only stretch to sixty-five degrees. Then, when you move the joint past sixty-five degrees, the scar tissue tears away from the normal tissue, and because scar tissue has more pain fibers, this is really going to hurt! And now you have another injury that is going to be repaired with even more scar tissue and probably with more restrictions of motion.

Physical therapy can help scar tissue with a technique known as remodeling, which involves breaking up old deposits of scar tissue that have formed in patterns that are not consistent with the direction in which the normal tissue fibers are aligned. With the remodeling process, the old scar tissue is broken down, and the new tissue is modeled to go in the same direction as the normal fibers, thereby increasing flexibility and limiting the chance of further tearing.

Orthopedic Surgery

Sometimes physical therapy isn't going to work, and you really need to see an orthopedic surgeon. Some injuries immediately require surgery because the damage is so significant that there is no other option. On the other hand, the problem may be so chronic and advanced that calcium deposits, bone spurs, torn tendons or ligaments, or cartilage degeneration make any kind of recovery impossible without surgical intervention. That doesn't mean that any of the therapies previously described won't have a place in a surgery patient's future, but before any of them can be effective, the damage is going to have to be resolved.

While it's unfortunate that some people really have suffered permanent physical damage to some part of their bodies, this is not the case for most of us. This means there's a great deal of hope that the rest of us really can resolve our pain and learn how to keep our bodies healthy.

Actually resolving pain syndromes requires more effort and commitment than just reaching for another bottle of pills; and simply masking symptoms has far-reaching health consequences that must be considered. It's not only about how you feel today, but about how you will age and what you will have to look forward to as you age. So if you're experiencing pain of any kind, I implore you to try any or all of the therapies I have discussed and to not give up. If you persist, you will most likely make that pain go away, not by masking symptoms, but by treating the cause.

Richard Weinstein, D.C.

THE NOT-SO-COMMON COMMONSENSE DIET

You're Actually Going to Put That in Your Mouth?

Following the triangle of health with its framework of structural, chemical, and mental/emotional integrity, it's time to explore the chemical component. This whole topic can be simplified by breaking it down into those things we put into our bodies that help us, and those things that hurt us.

It's been said that nothing is so uncommon as common sense, and I can think of nothing more appropriate than this statement when considering all the controversy concerning what constitutes a proper diet. The American obsession regarding diet would be hysterically funny were it not for the tragedy of so many people hurting themselves by chasing one crazy diet plan after another. The laughter really stops when we finally grasp just how seriously we're damaging ourselves by the food choices we make on a daily basis.

In Search of the Magic Diet

Thanks to weight-loss programs, diet gurus, and diet-of-the-week fads, the US diet business has become a **sixty billion dollar** industry as people continually search for the magic diet. We've got protein diets, low-carbohydrate diets, grapefruit diets, diets based on your blood type, rotation diets, liquid diets—basically everything except common sense and personal responsibility diets.

Let me just state that if you're significantly overweight it's either because you're eating processed foods and fast foods that cause hormonal imbalances, have an unhealthy emotional relationship with food, a hormonal imbalance, or a combination of these factors. Keep in mind that in the human body, one problem can lead to another, which in turn exacerbates the original problem. This is often the case with diet and hormones, and once again fits the vicious cycle model.

First and foremost, we have to stop pretending that there is some magical diet plan that requires no responsibility on our part and that will make us as slim as some genetically-blessed model. We also have to stop thinking that the subject of diet is as complicated as rocket science, because it simply isn't. What is a reasonable diet is painfully obvious, but for a variety of reasons most people rebel and eat all kinds of garbage.

Without launching into a sociological essay on human behavior, I think the four primary reasons why people eat such an array of unhealthy foods and have such unbalanced diets are:

1. They are conditioned to have an emotional attachment to certain foods.

2. The vast majority of fast foods and processed foods contain glutamate—which is very different from glutamine—purposely added to them by food manufacturers because it's highly addictive, and incidentally causes hormonal imbalances.

3. They are bombarded by the relentless advertising and marketing campaigns of the manufacturers of these foods (and I use the term loosely here).

4. They have hormonal imbalances.

Unfortunately, all four factors are usually interrelated, and together they perpetuate an unhealthy eating cycle.

Richard Weinstein, D.C.

Why a Good Diet isn't Rocket Science

Let's see just how complex and difficult it is to have a good diet.

The human body requires good-quality proteins, carbohydrates, and essential fatty acids to function properly. Since eating is nothing more or less than a refueling of nutrients on a regular basis, it's logical that we should eat good-quality proteins, carbohydrates, and fats in reasonable quantities at each and every meal.

Where in the world we ever got the idea that each meal should be different in its nutritional content is beyond understanding, but in the case of breakfast, I have a strong suspicion that the cereal and bread manufacturers had a lot to do with it.

When you wake up in the morning, your blood sugar is going to be low because you probably haven't eaten anything for nine to twelve hours. It makes absolutely no sense to load your body up with nothing more substantial than a bunch of carbohydrates like cereal, toast, bagels, pastries, or waffles, and then wash it down with juice and caffeinated beverages. These are all foods that will rapidly convert into sugar and precipitate an insulin reaction that will cause you to have low blood sugar a couple of hours later. No wonder you're tired by ten o'clock in the morning and are looking for more sugar and caffeine to give you a jolt! You've also given yourself a great big dose of omega-6 fats, which cause systemic inflammation and cell wall receptor site dysfunction (described in Chapter 6).

For blood sugar stability, a good diet is no more complex than building a fire. To start a fire you need some paper and kindling (carbohydrates) because you need a fast-burning fuel to get things going. However, if at some point you don't start adding logs (protein) for a longer-lasting source of fuel, then either the fire is going to burn out or you will have to keep adding kindling frequently.

This is exactly what happens at breakfast for most people. They eat all kinds of carbohydrate foods that burn up quickly, leaving them tired, irritable, and craving more sugar. Or, even worse, if you plan your life so poorly that you don't have time for breakfast at all, which means you won't be breaking your fast until sometime around lunch time, you're basically running on empty until noon.

If you have children and are giving them juice, cereal, and a banana to start their day, is it any wonder they might have difficulty staying alert in class or have a tendency to become disruptive? Keep in mind that fruit juices are merely very concentrated amounts of sugar, and be aware that many fruit "juice" products can contain as little as 10 percent real juice while the rest of it is corn syrup and other additives. Even if it's real fruit juice, it might be natural sugar but sugar nonetheless. While most fruits can be very beneficial as a source of fiber, minerals, and vitamins, once you squeeze them into juice, you've lost the fiber and dramatically increased the sugar. When you consider how many oranges you can eat compared to how many you can drink, my point becomes obvious.

If your children begin their day with a carbohydrate high, their blood sugar will quickly begin its rapid descent. To add to the problem, it's pizza and a soda for lunch, with maybe a cookie, and there they go again. By the time these kids see something that resembles protein, it's dinnertime, and by then their blood sugar has been unbalanced throughout most of the day.

The Emotional/Hormonal Relationship with Food

Let's explore the emotional/hormonal relationship with food, and how emotions and hormones can work against each other and cause a lot of trouble.

When you were a little kid, what were you given if you behaved or did something well? What did your grandparents like to give you just because you were such a little darling? What was always present at holidays such as Halloween, Thanksgiving, Christmas, Easter, Valentine's Day, and birthdays? Sugar, and lots of it!! Cakes, pies, candy bars, chocolate bunnies, candy corn, heart-shaped candy, marshmallow peeps—you name it.

It's not hard to imagine how we learned to associate sugar with fun, parties, affection, and reward. We became conditioned to love sugar because it represents positive emotions; it tastes good; and it gives us a short-term glucose high. Looked at in a certain context, it's our first experience with mind-altering substances, and when eaten without enough protein to stabilize blood sugar levels, it becomes addictive.

The more sugar you consume, the more insulin your pancreas secretes. Insulin is responsible for enabling sugar to enter the liver, where it will be enzymatically converted into usable glucose or stored as glycogen.

It takes time for the liver to make this conversion; in the meantime the blood sugar level in the body will be low because the insulin has pulled the sugar into the liver. Since the brain's primary fuel is sugar (glucose), the brain will demand that you eat more sugar when normal levels drop. So you eat more sugar and restart the cycle over and over again.

Perhaps when you were a little kid and your metabolism was more forgiving, or perhaps because you were running around and being physically active, you managed to stay in decent shape. But once you became an adult, a funny thing happened: you slowly but surely realized that you were gaining weight. Somehow that size six dress is now a size twelve, or the boxer shorts you wore in high school have become large enough to… Well, you get the point.

What happened?

What happened is that you unwittingly followed the exact program that ranchers use to fatten up farm animals: increased carbohydrate consumption. When you consume more carbohydrates than your body can use, your body **must** store it as fat. The excess carbohydrates cannot be excreted or eliminated through the urine, bowels, or in any other way. The idea here is that carbohydrates stored as fat can be reconverted to glucose in times of famine or extreme physical exertion.

Conversely, if you begin to exercise seriously and restrict your carbohydrate intake, the muscles that are being used will run out of glucose, forcing your body to convert the fat cells back into usable glucose. This is why a good exercise program is essential to weight loss. Unfortunately, if your cortisol levels are unbalanced, you still might not lose weight through exercising because cortisol can cause you to crave and eat more sugar, as well as hamper your ability to burn calories by slowing down your thyroid gland function.

Because appropriately restricting certain carbohydrates should help you lose weight, there are now diets that propose the elimination of all carbohydrates. The idea is to eat all the bacon, eggs, cheese, and steak you want. What could be more fun than that? Heck, you didn't like all of those vegetables your parents tried to make you eat when you were a kid anyway.

In all fairness, most diets that advocate a high quantity of protein do add carbohydrates after two or three weeks, but people often misinterpret the need for carbohydrates and think they will lose more weight if they simply stick with only eating protein.

The problem with eating mostly protein is that it can cause liver and kidney disorders, atherosclerosis (plaque in your arteries), and possibly diabetes. The absence of carbohydrates will mean a severe reduction in insulin, and if this occurs for a lengthy period of time, the liver will form substances called ketones and acetones that will harm the kidneys and liver.

So, you're still overweight and in search of the magical diet plan that will return your body to its glorious youth, unless you got a head start and became overweight as a child. You're resisting exercise because it takes up a lot of time and energy, and besides, you mow the lawn once a week and, in your mind, that should count for something. Not only that, but you work really hard, and your boss, spouse, and kids are driving you crazy, and you could use a little reward for being such a good person.

What could be better than an ultra-refined carbohydrate called alcohol to make those stresses go away? Or maybe a handful of M&M's or Hershey's Kisses? Haagen-Dazs anyone? Your daily diet doesn't support your blood sugar right from the start of your day, which makes you too tired to exercise, and you're cranky and so stressed out that your cortisol level is constantly pushing the reward button in your brain that says you not only need that candy bar but, by God, you **deserve** it! You've been conditioned to associate sugar with happiness and rewards; well, you could use a little happiness and reward.

The only problem is that the rewards are making you gain weight day after day, and that by itself is becoming pretty stressful. When you look in the mirror, you're not particularly proud of what you see, and soon you'll have to deal with your doctor warning you of the risks of heart problems and/or diabetes

With all this stress, what's a person to do? In all probability, you're going to respond to the need for immediate gratification and have another drink, candy bar, or ice cream cone, and decide that tomorrow will be the great day of change and reformation. Okay, maybe not tomorrow but certainly next week. Oh wait, that won't work because that's when your vacation, birthday, or the holidays are coming up and that wouldn't be a good time to start a diet…

Glutamate and Food Addictions

Back in the 1950s, fast food restaurants and processed food manufacturers learned to add glutamate to their products because it's a highly addictive substance that excites brain cells.

At first they used monosodium glutamate (MSG), but that created an obvious reaction in many people—everything from headaches to rashes, nausea, and fainting. Realizing that customers passing out or getting nauseous in your fast food restaurant really wasn't such a good selling point, they took out the monosodium and left in the glutamate, which is really the addictive ingredient anyway. The joke among these food merchants is that the glutamate builds "brand loyalty," which is a euphemism for "addiction."

Amazingly, no one thought it was funny when cigarette companies put addictive chemicals in their product, but food companies get away with it with the blessing of the Food and Drug Administration (FDA). As far as the FDA is concerned, if MSG in put into a food product, the company has to list it as such on the label. But if it's just the glutamate that's been added, not only do they not have to put it on the label, but they can hide it by calling it hydrolyzed protein, soy extract, yeast, and—worst of all—natural flavorings and natural seasonings.

Since glutamate is a protein amino acid made in the body from L-glutamate, the FDA says it's natural. However, your body knows exactly how much glutamate to make and never makes more than what is needed, which means there's no barrier to stop it going directly to your brain. So whatever amount of glutamate the food company puts in its product, it goes straight to your brain where it will excite the area of that is responsible for addictions. If fact, it can excite it so much that it can kill the cells, which is why glutamate is considered to be an **excitotoxin**.

If it wasn't bad enough that glutamate makes you addicted to foods high in inflammatory omega-6 oils (and by now you certainly know what all that means), the first thing that happens to lab animals given glutamate is that they get fat. This is because glutamate also kills the brain cells that manage hormone So now you have a whole new way to become hormonally unbalanced.

There are four things that have to happen if you're going to reverse the unhealthy cycle that results from the Standard American Diet (SAD):

- Have your cortisol levels checked with an ASI (adrenal stress index) test, and also have your insulin and glucose levels checked.

- Adopt a commonsense diet guided by knowledge regarding the foods you eat. Stop, and I mean **absolutely stop,** eating processed foods and fast foods that have glutamate snuck into them!

- Make a commitment to regular physical exercise.

- Arrive at a true understanding of your emotional/psychological relationship with food and decide that you don't want to be a pawn for every clever advertisement that promises you thrills, fun, or sex, because you consume their beer, burgers, or soda.

It's very important to reiterate that if your cortisol levels are unbalanced, and especially if the cause is intestinal inflammation, you will **not** get well, lose weight, or be able to keep your diet under control. If your cortisol levels are unbalanced, though you intellectually know you're doing all of the wrong things, and you even feel guilty about it, the cortisol will make you do them anyway.

It truly is sad to see some people try so hard and fail, when all that is wrong is their cortisol levels. Please get yours checked before you even bother with anything else, and refer to the previous chapter for ways to resolve these imbalances.

The following dietary recommendations are, of necessity, generalized; this means that this diet concept will work for most people most of the time. Just as I made the point at the beginning of this book that people respond to stress differently, it's difficult to find the one diet plan that will work for every single human being. If you have a specific illness or genetic disorder, then you should already be consulting with a nutritionist familiar with your special needs.

In the beginning of this chapter, I promised you that having a good diet did not have to be rocket science, and could be straightforward and easy to understand. I've found in my own practice that many people really do try to follow a good diet plan, but that some diets are so complicated and difficult to comprehend, with odd measurements and point systems, that they just give up and order a pizza with a diet soda.

The goal of any good diet is to have good-quality proteins, carbohydrates, and fats in appropriate amounts and in fixed ratios with each other. Let's take each food group in order and see how easy it is to incorporate them into a healthy, balanced diet.

Proteins

The first easy rule regarding proteins comes from the National Research Council, which recommends that you calculate your daily protein requirement in grams by taking your weight in pounds and dividing it by two. This means that if you weigh 140 pounds, then you will need 70 grams of protein per day. If you're very physically active you may require a little more, and if you're trying to lose weight by increasing your level of exercise, then you won't.

The second easy rule about proteins and grams is that per ounce, all meat proteins are the same. This means that chicken, beef, pork, lamb, or turkey all average 7 grams of protein per ounce. Conveniently, one egg equals 7 grams of protein. Even fish is pretty close to this average, with a range of 5 to 7 grams of protein per ounce.

So if you require 70 grams of protein per day, you can have 10 ounces of meat or fish daily, or 8 ounces if you have two eggs for breakfast. Since this is supposed to be a commonsense diet, it presumes you will choose lean cuts of meat that are not loaded with fat and not assume that pork means bacon or sausage.

A lot of people get a little testy about how they're supposed to know how many ounces a piece of meat or fish weighs without getting their old kitchen scale out. Fortunately, we live in such a great country that it's nearly impossible to buy any protein in a market that does not have the weight listed right on the package.

Let's say you go to the market and buy a package of four skinless chicken breasts for dinner that total a pound. This would mean that each chicken breast weighs 4 ounces (and contains 28 [4x7] grams of protein), so you still need six more ounces (or 42 grams) of protein to meet your daily requirement—in this example, 70 grams. For lunch you grab a can of tuna, and the label tells you it weighs 6 ounces. If you eat half of the can (3x7=21), you still have three more ounces (21g) of protein to go. This means that for breakfast you could have two eggs and get very close to your total protein requirement. In reality, you will probably get there easily because there will be a few grams of protein in the bread you're likely to put the tuna on or in the toast you have with your eggs.

There are also other types of protein that are going to be in your diet, and you need to know how to figure them into how much you may consume. Somehow, with proteins, seven seems to be the lucky number. One cup of milk or yogurt equals 7 grams of protein. A half cup of beans or legumes (such as split peas or lentils) equals 7 grams of protein, as does an ounce of almonds, peanuts, or tofu.

So if you pay just a little attention to the weight of the protein foods you're buying, you should have very little difficulty figuring out how much you should eat. You can also make it less difficult by buying in quantities that are easy to calculate. Instead of buying two-thirds of a pound of lunch meat, buy either a half or a whole pound.

Carbohydrates

Unlike its guidelines for proteins, the National Research Council has no specific daily requirements for how many carbohydrates an individual should consume. This is the part of the diet that people struggle with most, both in terms of which kinds and how many carbohydrates they should be eating.

In order to make intelligent choices about which carbohydrates you should eat, you need to be aware that not all carbohydrates are absorbed the same way. Some are more quickly digested and the resulting sugars released more rapidly into the bloodstream. A particular carbohydrate's ability to raise blood sugar levels is assigned a numerical value called the *glycemic index*. The carbohydrates that have the highest numerical value on the glycemic index are the ones that will cause the greatest output of insulin and thus lead to weight gain, fatigue, and increased carbohydrate cravings.

Carbohydrates that enter the bloodstream very quickly and raise blood sugar levels abruptly will cause an elevated insulin response, which in turn will actually result in low blood sugar as the excess insulin performs its task of whisking the sugar off to the liver to be processed into glucose. At this point, the low blood sugar will make you crave more sugar, and you restart the negative cycle all over again. Keep in mind that any sugar your body doesn't burn up with activity gets stored away as fat for future use.

Now I could torture you with an extensive list of the glycemic index of every known carbohydrate, but that simply isn't necessary; instead, I'm just going to give you a short list so you get an idea about how it works:

NO WONDER YOU FEEL LIKE CRAP!

Glycemic Index of Common Foods

Apples	39	Pears	38
Bagel	72	Pizza	80
Baked potato	111	(plain baked dough	
Banana	62	with parmesan cheese	
Brown rice	50	and tomato sauce)	
Cashews	27	Skim milk	32
Carrots	35	Sweet potato	61
Corn tortilla	52	Watermelon	72
Grapes	59	White rice	89
Green peas	51	White Bread	72
Honey	61	Whole milk	41
Lentils	29	Whole wheat	72
Navy beans	31	bread	
Oranges	40	Yogurt (low fat)	27

It'll be a lot easier if we just think in terms of "best" or "helpful" carbohydrates and "unhelpful" or "second best" ones.

The "unhelpful" carbohydrates are bread, pasta, grains, potatoes, corn, cereals, rice and rice cakes, papayas, bananas, raisins and other dried fruits, and most fruit juices. Does this mean you're never going to eat them again? Of course not. But it does mean that you should eat them less frequently and in smaller amounts.

The "helpful" carbohydrates are obviously everything else that's left, but even then, some are better than others.

In the following lists we'll divide the rest of the carbohydrates into two groups; the first group contains the ones that will affect your blood sugar levels the least, and those will be the carbohydrates that you want to eat the most; the second group contains the carbohydrates you may still eat, but in moderation.

Richard Weinstein, D.C.

Best Carbohydrates

- Apple
- Apricots
- Artichoke
- Asparagus
- Bean sprouts
- Black beans
- Blueberries
- Bok Choy
- Broccoli
- Brussels sprouts
- Cabbage
- Cauliflower
- Celery
- Cherries
- Collard greens
- Cucumber
- Eggplant
- Endive
- Grapefruit
- Green beans
- Kale
- Kidney beans
- Kiwi
- Leeks
- Lentils
- Lettuce (not iceberg)
- Mushrooms
- Nectarine
- Okra
- Onions
- Orange
- Peach
- Pear
- Peppers
- Pineapple
- Radishes
- Spinach
- Swiss chard
- Tangerine
- Tomato
- Turnip
- Yellow squash
- Zucchini

Second-Best Carbohydrates

- Acorn squash
- Beets
- Butternut squash
- Carrots
- Lima beans
- Parsnip
- Peas
- Sweet potato

Perhaps you've noticed the glaring absence of certain carbohydrates, such as, corn, potatoes, rice, pasta, bread, and baked goods. The reason for this is that in an ideal diet, you want to avoid these carbohydrates, because they're all very high on the glycemic index, and in the case of corn, potatoes, and pasta, they can increase systemic inflammation. Again, this doesn't mean you can never eat corn on the cob or a baked potato again, just go easy and don't make them staples of your diet.

Getting Beat by Wheat (Gluten)

Since this book was first published we've seen a dramatic problem caused by the way most of our wheat is grown, and one that's certainly caused a great deal of hormonal imbalances and health issues. While our wheat hasn't technically been genetically modified, it's been hybridized into a strain that isn't compatible for many people.

About six years ago, just when I thought I had the whole cortisol / inflammation / intestinal tract / hormonal imbalance problem figured out, all of a sudden patients began showing up with the same type of hormone problems, except that now they weren't responding as well to the 3R Program. There was no logical explanation for this until a research study funded by the Australian National Health and Medical Research Council discovered that the nearly endless genetic modification and hybridization of wheat has created a gluten protein that is a poor match for many peoples' genes, with some disastrous results. Rye and barley also have this problem, and oats that have been stored near this type of wheat have been contaminated with this gluten protein, too.

There are two genetic mismatches for this type of wheat. The first one causes intestinal tract inflammation, and if you've gotten this far in this book, you know exactly what that means.

The genetic inability to digest gluten is called celiac disease, and today's new version of this is called pseudo-celiac disease. The initial symptoms are bloating after eating the gluten and—for many—joint pain and fatigue. It's estimated that at least forty percent of the population is sensitive to this new gluten, and all you need to do to realize the scale of this problem is go to the grocery store and see how many gluten-free products are now available.

The next genetic mismatch is far scarier because it triggers an autoimmune attack on your brain. It's called **gluten ataxia** or **gluten encephalopathy**, and the scary part of the problem is that you don't know if you have it until parts of your brain are damaged enough to cause symptoms, for which there is absolutely no treatment. Symptoms of gluten encephalopathy include migraine headaches, dizziness, difficulty speaking, visual difficulties, and loss of control of arms or legs. Seizures can also be a part of this symptom complex. There is a Mayo clinic study that shows brain pathology found by postmortem examination to be directly associated with gluten exposure.

Another problem with this gluten is that it will cause some people to make a form of morphine out of it in their brain, called gluteomorphine. This will cause you to crave gluten products because they're literally making you high. In my office this becomes fairly evident when I ask a patient I suspect of suffering this problem what their favorite foods are, and they answer pasta, pizza, macaroni and cheese, and grilled cheese sandwiches. Another way to tell is to have them stop eating all gluten for two weeks. What happens is that they go through morphine withdrawal and are very irritable and cranky. The best way to positively identify this problem is to test through the Cyrex Lab gluten sensitivity panel which tests for two types of gluteomorphines; you will find Cyrex in the Resources Guide.

Unfortunately, we're still not done with the gluten problem, and here's where it really confused me at first.

The 3R Program I use to help restore thyroid function was going right off the tracks and had virtually stopped working. What used to be rather straightforward became impossible-to get-results with, until the discovery that today's gluten molecules look just like thyroid tissue to the body's defenses and thus provoke an autoimmune attack on the thyroid gland. So as long as the patient was eating gluten, the autoimmune issues just got worse. It's therefore imperative that all thyroid patients stop eating gluten. Recent research also shows that a similar phenomenon is occurring with gluten causing an autoimmune attack on the pancreas cells that secrete insulin, causing what is now called Latent Autoimmune Diabetes in Adults (LADA).

I'm fully aware that many people don't believe there is anything wrong with today's wheat/gluten products, and it's mostly those who are genetically lucky enough to not to be affected by eating it (of course, they might also be in line for getting the horrendous symptoms of gluten encephalopathy but just haven't gotten there yet). Other sceptics think it's just a way of ascribing health problems to some esoteric "problem" called gluten sensitivity. If you are one of those readers, I invite you to go to the References section at the end of the book and check out the research sources regarding gluten.

Most gluten-free products are made with rice flour, and today you can find gluten-free bread, pasta, pizza dough, pie crust, bagels, and on and on. While this is something of a help, let's still remember that this is still a poor choice in carbohydrates any way you turn it around. In what I find to be perhaps the most absurd example of just how bad all this has become and how the market for gluten-free products has become a financial boon, you can now buy a nitrate-filled, carcinogenic hot dog on a gluten-free bun in many Major League Baseball parks!

When Bobby entered my office he was nine years old and he couldn't remember a single day in his life when his stomach didn't hurt. He would experience pain at varying levels and it would often prevent him from going to school and participating in other activities. He had been evaluated and treated by a host of doctors, including a pediatric gastroenterologist from Stanford, and had been taking an acid-blocking drug (prilosec) for over two years with no change in symptoms. The Stanford doctor insisted that he didn't have any sensitivity or allergy to wheat or gluten based on a blood test that only checked for one antibody.

When I asked him what his favorite foods were, he told me they were macaroni and cheese, pizza, and grilled cheese sandwiches. I told his mother that he most likely has a problem with wheat gluten but she at first was adamant that she didn't want to keep him away from his favorite foods. So I tried the 3R Program with him with minimal results, and then I insisted we run the Cyrex Lab panel for gluten sensitivity, which tests for twenty-four different antibodies and two types of gluteomorphine.

The lab results showed that Bobby had 9 positive antibodies to gluten and tested positive to both gluteomorphines, which clearly explained why he liked wheat-based foods so much. With this conclusive evidence, he and his mother agreed to get him off all gluten products, and we kept up with the 3R Program and stopped the prilosec.

He came back in three weeks and reported that he was 80% better, and this surprised his mother because she thought he was doing even better than that. By the end of the visit he confessed that yes, he was actually better than that, but that he was having a little trouble with the fact that he couldn't use his stomach aches to get out of going to school. So I told him to come back in another three weeks when the school year was over, and he was 100% better.

*Epilogue: the Stanford doctor disputed the lab results because they weren't done by **his** lab, and was completely unfazed by this young man's recovery after nine long years of pain.*

Proteins and Carbohydrates Together

Now that we've established a hierarchy of carbohydrates, we need to determine how much you can eat to maintain a balance with your protein consumption.

If you're eating from the Best Carbohydrate list, then a good rule of thumb is to have twice as much carbohydrate as protein. You can usually do this with a simple visual assessment. When you also consider that all the "helpful" carbohydrates are loaded with fiber, vitamins, and minerals, it really is hard to eat too much to the point where it would be detrimental to your health.

When determining the amount of second-best or "unhelpful" carbohydrates to consume, you want to keep the ratios even, so that the amount of carbohydrate appears to be about the same as the amount of protein. For example, if you're having half a chicken breast, then half a baked potato would look about right. A mound of rice or rice pasta that is the same size as the protein serving would be okay.

You also want to make sure that you don't have two "unhelpful" carbohydrates in the same meal. You don't want to combine corn, carrots, beets, potatoes, rice, or pasta because they will overload the glycemic index of the meal. A classic example of this is

Thanksgiving dinner, when sweet potatoes, bread stuffing, mashed potatoes, glazed carrots, and pumpkin pie conspire to create a disastrous blood sugar crescendo and leave the participants lying semiconscious on the sofa. So the best choice you can make when putting a meal together is to have a reasonable amount of lean protein with good, fresh vegetables or fruits from the "helpful" carbohydrate list.

The sticking point in this program for most people has to do with bread and what to eat for breakfast. It isn't too difficult to figure out what to eat for dinner if you're choosing the correct amounts of chicken, fish, beef, pork, or tofu with "helpful" carbohydrates. Even lunch isn't too challenging if you choose a sandwich of gluten-free bread with a good amount of protein, lettuce and tomato, a hearty soup, or a salad with protein in it. But we've become so conditioned to a carbohydrate-laden breakfast that it's difficult to figure out what type of protein sounds appealing first thing in the morning.

One obvious choice would be eggs, and an option for those who are either pressed for time or don't function terribly well in the early morning is to make several hard boiled eggs ahead of time to have on hand. Other good choices include cottage cheese or yogurt. Ideally, you want to stay with plain yogurt and add your own fruit because the fruit preserves in yogurt are loaded with sugar. A slice of gluten-free bread with natural peanut butter (make sure it's not the typical grocery-store variety with hydrogenated oils and sugar added to it). Almond butter is another option.

My favorite recommendation to the time-challenged/don't-knowwhat-to-eat-for-breakfast person is a protein drink. Protein powders can be bought in any health food store (many grocery stores also sell them), and they can be made from egg whites, whey, or soy. They can be strictly protein or they can also contain carbohydrates, which really makes them a complete meal. How you decide which one to purchase depends on what you plan to mix it with. If you're going to mix the powder with water or milk, you'll want the kind with carbohydrates added in order to keep your nutrients balanced; if you're going to add fruit or fruit juice to it, then you might want to stick to the protein-only powder. My advice is to use a blender and make a quart at a time to store in the refrigerator. That way you won't be washing the blender every day, and it will be conveniently waiting for you in the morning. Just drink it and go—no muss, no fuss.

Fats

This is the really easy part once you put the onion dip away.

Your body does need essential fatty acids to function normally, and the best way to get these is from fish. Other than that, you should use only olive oil, unless you absolutely have to deep-fry something, and then I would recommend soybean or peanut oil. Olive oil is an anti-inflammatory omega 9 oil and has been shown to relieve pain just as well as aspirin. You do not want to use canola or vegetable oils, and you do want to learn how to make your own salad dressing and avoid the store-bought varieties. If you cannot find the time to whisk together some olive oil, vinegar, and herbs, then you need to reassess your life.

The topic of omega-6 versus omega-3 fats has recently become enormously important in medical research because of the far-reaching health problems related to excessive dietary omega-6 fats. If you recall Chapter 3, omega-6 oils cause inflammation by making highly inflammatory chemicals. The omega-6 fats, which come from corn oil, hydrogenated oils, fatty meats, most baked goods, margarine, and deep-fried foods, have been scientifically linked to coronary heart disease and elevated cholesterol, atherosclerosis, thrombosis, systemic inflammation, Alzheimer's disease, rheumatoid arthritis and other autoimmune disorders, as well as receptor site dysfunction that inhibits neurotransmitter attachment to the cell membrane, which in turn can result in psychiatric disorders and hormonal imbalances.

Given the fact that the American diet is loaded with omega-6 oils (on any given day in the United States about one-quarter of the adult population visits a fast-food restaurant, and Americans spend more than $110 billion a year on fast food, which is more than they spend on movies, books, magazines, newspapers, videos, and recorded music combined), is it any wonder we're one of the sickest nations on the planet?

Because of my obvious and longstanding concern regarding inflammation and its effect on human health, I find the current interest and research into inflammation fascinating; I also see an inevitable and ugly showdown looming in the future. It's like two huge trains on the same track heading toward each other: One train is bona fide medical research, and the other is the fast food industry, which includes the soft drink industry. This pits solid research that says this junk food is making us sick and even psychiatrically disturbed against giants such as McDonalds, Burger King, Coca-Cola, and Pepsi. Watch this space.

Beyond the obvious need to avoid foods that are high in omega-6 oils, the cure to all this lies in actively consuming omega-3 oils, which are found in pumpkin seeds, walnuts, beans, soy products, and, most significantly, fish and fish oils. Most research indicates that omega-3 from fish oil is easily assimilated in the body. Omega-3 oils protect the vascular system, reduce inflammation in the brain, have a specific role in brain development and regeneration of nerve cells, reduce the risk of coronary heart disease and cardiac arrhythmia, relieve the pain and swelling of rheumatoid arthritis, and inhibit autoimmune reactions.

While there is no known RDA (recommended daily allowance) for omega-3 oils, research studies on rheumatoid arthritis used doses of 1,500 mg with good results. If you have a good diet, a daily dose of 1,000 mg per day seems like a reasonable amount. If your diet isn't too wonderful just yet, or you're at risk of heart disease or depression, you might want to go as high as 4,000 mg per day. Recent research indicates that an increase in omega-3 oils might result in a depletion of antioxidants in the body, so it's important to take antioxidant vitamins when taking omega-3 oils. Antioxidants are so essential to human health, you should be taking them anyway. The antioxidant vitamins are E, A, C, and grape seed extract; I'll go into further detail on this subject later in this chapter.

Other good sources of fat are avocados, tahini (sesame seed butter), and raw nuts. When necessary, you should **always** use butter instead of margarine, since one is actually a food and the other is not.

Which brings us to our next category.

Things You Shouldn't Put in Your Mouth

Remarkably, human beings eat all kinds of garbage that can't even be classified as food, and about 90 percent of the money Americans spend on food is used to buy processed food.

What exactly is the nutritional value of coffee or soda? Zero would be the correct answer. And what of "foods" that have been so over-processed as to be devoid of any nutritional benefit, such as potato chips, cheese puffs, fast foods, and lots of wonderful convenience foods found in your supermarket's freezer whose ingredients would require that you have a degree in chemistry in order to figure out what they actually are? Beyond the problem of the omega-6 oils and inflammation previously discussed, there are other reasons to avoid processed and fast foods.

Excitotoxins are substances like glutamate (not to be confused with glutamine), *aspartame*, and cysteine, which are commonly used as flavor enhancers (e.g., monosodium glutamate or MSG), and artificial sweeteners.

In labeling foods, manufacturers always disguise Excitotoxins under lots of other names including "hydrolyzed protein" and, worse, "natural flavorings" and "natural seasonings." The Food and Drug Administration (FDA) is fully aware of the dangers of glutamate and has known so since the 1950's, but clearly they have no appetite for a fight with the processed and fast food giants. From their point of view, since glutamate is a naturally occurring amino acid converted selectively by your body from glutamine, it passes muster as a "natural" substance.

The difference is that your body knows how much glutamate to make to stimulate your brain, so there is no barrier to stop glutamate going to your brain. But when it's crammed into so many of the foods you may be eating, that extra glutamate travels up to your brain, excites the addictive center, and ultimately excites the brain cells to death. The companies that put this stuff in their products do so because they know it will make you addicted to it, and they jokingly refer to it as creating "brand loyalty." A minor problem is that it also kills the hormonal cells in the brain, and when they give it to lab animals the animals become fat.

The human body is a dynamic masterpiece of chemical interactions, and how we've come to a place where we routinely put all manner of toxic trash into our bodies is completely beyond comprehension. Earlier in this chapter I noted the many different types of diets that are based on so many conflicting rationales. Most of these diets do have one thing in common as far as weight loss is concerned and that is that they only work **if the dieter doesn't have the hormonal imbalances I've been telling you about.** The reason for this is that they all share a common thread, which is the avoidance of processed and refined foods. It's as simple as that! This is a good reason to avoid the low-calorie frozen meals offered by some weight-loss companies, for while they might be low in calories, they usually contain glutamate and a lot of other artificial ingredients.

Whether it's the Atkins low-carbohydrate/high-protein diet, or the Zone 40-30-30 (ratio of carbohydrates to protein to fats) diet, or the Eat Right for Your Type (a different diet for different blood types) diet, or the McDougall high-carbohydrate/low-protein diet, they all forbid junk food. All of these diets eliminate refined flours, refined sugars, hydrogenated oils, and food additives and preservatives. By doing away with all of this garbage and eating real food in reasonable amounts, people are bound to lose weight.

The next thing you should never put in your mouth is high fructose corn syrup (HFCS). HFCS is twice as sweet as regular cane sugar, but your body can't break it down like regular sugar. In fact, your pancreas won't even secret insulin for HFCS, so it goes directly to your liver where it's converted into fat.

Think about this for a moment. Every single time you eat or drink something with HFCS you're adding more fat to your body! HFCS is in everything from sodas, caffeinated energy drinks, cereals, juices, jams and jellies, pasta and ravioli meals, peanut butter—well, you get the point: it's in everything imaginable. At least the FDA makes them put it on the label so you can easily avoid it.

Last, but certainly not least, is soda, and there are several reasons to avoid putting this in your mouth. Soda is very high on the list of causative factors for the rise in obesity and diabetes. In 1944 the average amount of soda per person was 90 eight ounce servings a year; by 2000 it increased to **600 servings** a year. Today a twelve-ounce soda has between forty and fifty grams of HFCS which equals **10 teaspoons** of sugar and 150 calories that turn immediately to fat. At that rate, just one soda a day will cause you to gain about 15 pounds a year.

Another two problems with soda are related to either the phosphoric acid or citric acids in them. The first problem is that these acids can cause intestinal tract inflammation; the second is that they dramatically alter your blood pH to such a level of acidity that your body has to pour calcium into your bloodstream to balance it back out, and the calcium is coming out of your bones! This is why today's teenagers are expected to have high rates of osteoporosis considering how much soda they drink.

Now that you know which foods can help you and which ones can sabotage your efforts to have a diet that is nutritionally and hormonally supportive, here comes the commonsense part.

Food as Fuel

The concept that you really need to embrace is that eating represents a fuel-delivery system to your body. It's not enough to stuff any old thing into your stomach to relieve the sensation of hunger; the goal is to provide your body with the correct balance of nutrients that'll keep you healthy and vital every single day. Unfortunately, most people don't approach their diets this way, even though they intellectually know better.

For a useful analogy, compare your need for fuel to that of your car. When your body's getting low on fuel your brain creates the sensation of hunger, which triggers the desire for food. With regard to your stomach, you're trying to go from empty to full. Your car's fuel gauge does the same thing, but instead of the physical sensations that let you know when it's time to refuel, there's a gauge to make you aware of the level of gas in the tank.

So let's say it's time to rush off to work and, *oops!* your car's fuel gauge reads very close to empty and you'll run out of gas before you get to work. You're going to have to take some action to bring the gauge from empty to full. Well, maybe you don't really have the time to drive to the gas station, so why not grab the garden hose and fill the tank with water? Or you could run back into the house and get a couple of half gallons of soda and pour them into the tank. Either way you're adding fluid to a gauge that measures liquid content, and if you turn the ignition key to just the place where the electrical system engages, you're going to see the needle go from E (empty) to F (full). Mission accomplished!

What's that you say? This is the stupidest thing you've ever heard of, because putting any old liquid into the fuel tank will destroy the engine and render the car useless?

This is no different to dumping some sugar-coated product and a cup of coffee into your stomach to create the sensation of "full" and thinking that you're going to end up in any better condition than your car will. The only difference is that your car will die immediately, whereas your body will let you get away with this foolishness for a while. And while you can always buy another car, it's not likely that science will advance to the point that you can buy another body in the near future.

The commonsense approach to a healthy diet is to ask yourself a very simple basic question, "Is this going to be good for me or bad for me?" Is the next thing you put in your mouth going to represent usable fuel or just a bunch of toxins your liver is going to have to figure out how to get rid of? Does putting a particular substance into your stomach make any sense, or is it just as stupid as putting water or soda into your car's gas tank?

As straightforward and simplistic as all this may sound, at the heart of the problem are the intangible quirks of human nature: it's usually easier to lie to ourselves that one more day of a bad diet won't matter, and immediate gratification supersedes long-range common sense.

Recent research proves that we're hardwired for short-term reward over long-term benefit, although at the same time we're quite capable of planning for long-term projects that benefit us. So a good approach to handling these competing drives is to regard your diet, and therefore your health, as a long-term project that you become committed to. The same mind that can conceive of and build a skyscraper or get us to the moon can also navigate through life with a conscious awareness of what constitutes good food.

As a daily reminder of why a healthy diet is a good idea, you could vividly imagine what you'll look and feel like if you keep eating garbage day after day, year after year into the future. To this end, start noticing the elderly people you encounter in the grocery store, the mall, or the bank. Some of them will be fit and vital, physically capable of leading active lives, while others will be so overweight and in such poor condition that they use the grocery cart as a walker.

While I realize that there are a several other factors (e.g., genetics, injury, and diseases) in addition to diet that influence how we'll age, diet is the one factor we have control of most of the time.

There are instances, however, when we're not in control.

Hormone Imbalances Cause Food Cravings

I know I may have sounded harsh with this commonsense and personal responsibility perspective, so it's time for a little sympathy.

The dynamics of how people gain weight remain consistent, but what initiates the dynamic varies. For some it can be that they've developed an unhealthy psychological relationship to food and are using it as a crutch; for others it can be that they just got unlucky with an injury or a disease that caused them to take long-term NSAIDs or antibiotics, which resulted in the leaky gut/high-cortisol syndrome and blood sugar imbalances. In either case, whether the stress hormones are psychologically or physiologically induced, the food cravings that result are very real.

As I've already mentioned, stress hormones dominate the brain chemicals of rational thought. So even though you **know** that candy bar isn't going to make you feel or look any better, if your hormones are unbalanced, you will be driven to eat it. This is what happens to people who attempt to faithfully follow diet programs but find themselves cheating or, worse, find that they don't lose much weight because their hormonal metabolic rate will not cooperate. By following the program discussed in Chapter 6 on how to correct hormone imbalances, you'll be able to regain hormone stability so that you can be in control of what you choose to eat.

Another point that I want to make is that we're not expecting to achieve sainthood with regard to our diet; we're seeking balance and good health. Does this mean you'll never have an ice cream cone, a martini, or a bonbon again? Of course not! What it means is that you'll consume food responsibly with a conscious awareness of the nutrients you're fueling your body with most of the time. If your diet is good eighty-five percent of the time, you can certainly allow yourself to indulge in the occasional treat—just make sure it's not on the list of things to never put in your mouth. Go for high quality dark chocolate, or a really good quality ice cream with only natural ingredients. The problems occur when over half of the stuff you consume hardly even qualifies as nutritious food (such as meals from fast-food restaurants), or when the food choices you make are so unbalanced they compromise your internal chemistry

The Pro-Inflammatory State and Dietary Factors in Pain

There are three reasons why a good diet is pertinent to this discussion of cortisol imbalances.

A poor diet can cause: (i) spinal and peripheral joint pain; (ii) hormonal imbalances; and (iii) leaky gut syndrome. As we have seen in the previous chapters, these three problems can be intimately related and perpetuate each other.

There isn't a chiropractor or medical doctor in the world who hasn't encountered patients in severe pain who insist that there was no physical activity on their part that would cause that level of suffering. They didn't lift anything; they weren't gardening or washing the car; they weren't even bending over and reaching for something. Their stress levels are fine, and they weren't even thinking evil thoughts. But suddenly, out of the blue, their back went into spasm and now they can barely move.

This is the time for the doctor to ask the patient what he or she has been eating, because dietary imbalances can cause the body to go into the pro-inflammatory state of systemic inflammation, which can cause irritation of the pain neurons inside the joints. The term "pro-inflammatory state" describes an increase in substances that exist naturally in the body but which become chemical irritants at excessively high levels.

A diet that's deficient in certain vitamins or minerals can result in an excess of these chemical irritants. Similarly, a diet that's too high in fats, caffeine, and toxins will also cause an increase in pro-inflammatory chemicals. The pro-inflammatory state is characterized by increased tissue acidity, increased free radicals, fatty-acid imbalance, and insufficient mineral intake (particularly potassium).

What happens is that a poor diet elevates levels of these substances to the point where they irritate the pain nerve fibers inside of the joints, which in turn will trigger intense muscle spasms. The muscle spasms then further distort the alignment of the joint, meaning that they restrict the ability of the joint to move in its normal manner, which further irritates the nerves in the joint. It's another one of those vicious cycles in which things go from bad to worse.

A good example (something that I see several times a year in my practice) involves the inflammatory chemical arachidonic acid. Foods that contain arachidonic acid are beef, pork, lamb, dairy, shrimp, lobster, clams, and, worst of all, hydrogenated oils/trans fats. I live and practice on the California coast, where there's a propensity toward seafood consumption. So every now and then when I get patients who have intense back pain and can't think of a single reason for it, I amaze them with my psychic skills by asking them if they've been eating a lot of shellfish lately. They look at me with astonishment and then go on to tell me that their market was having a great sale on shrimp or prawns and that they've been eating them for days.

The omega-3 oils in the 3R Program help to balance arachidonic acid levels.

Free Radicals

The next factor in the pro-inflammatory state is free radicals.

A free radical consists of an atom or group of atoms (molecule) with an unpaired electron. Free radicals work like a game of musical chairs, in which the last person left standing when the music stops is the loser. In the game of free radical musical chairs, the atom that's left unpaired attempts to disturb the molecular balance of the other atoms.

Free radicals damage protein molecules, DNA, and the protective fat barrier containing the receptor sites that surround each cell. They've been linked to many diseases, including cancer, but they're also a normal by-product of digestion.

The body's ability to rid itself of free radicals depends on another group of chemicals called antioxidants, and problems can occur if there are too many free radicals. In a research article titled "The Support for a Role for Antioxidants in Reducing Cancer," the author, G. Block, states: "Without continuous and abundant antioxidant and radical scavenging capability, survival would be impossible."

From the perspective of diet, the greatest risk of high levels of free radicals comes from eating processed foods that contain all kinds of chemicals that have nothing to do with nutrition. These chemicals are used for the manufacturer's benefit to hold the product together, enhance its shelf life, or affect its color, texture, or taste. But in your body they are toxins that your liver is going to have to work hard to get rid of.

The danger is that these free radicals can disrupt the normal molecular arrangement of your cells and cause them to malfunction. In terms of pain, free radicals irritate joints and soft tissues such as muscles and ligaments. This is why you're taking curcumin and resveratrol in the 3R Program.

Antioxidants

Antioxidants remove free radicals from the body. The most widely-known antioxidant is vitamin C, which performs many valuable functions. Vitamin C is essential in connective tissue repair, protects the body against infection, enhances the level of norepinephrine (the neurotransmitter the brain uses for alertness, concentration, and long-term memory formation), and is crucial for normal adrenal gland function—in fact, the adrenal glands use more vitamin C per gram of tissue than any other part of the body.

Foods rich in vitamin C are broccoli, citrus fruits, strawberries, celery, kiwi, tomatoes, peppers, and cantaloupe. Vitamin C supplements are easy to find, and a reasonable dosage would be 500 mg morning and night. Night-time supplementation of vitamin C can be especially important in recovering from an injury because the body repairs itself during sleep and uses vitamin C to repair connective tissue such as muscles, tendons, and ligaments.

The antioxidants known as *bioflavonoids* are so called because they occur in many of the same foods as vitamin C. Bioflavonoids are the compounds responsible for the color of some fruits and even some flowers. Research has shown that bioflavonoids protect cell membranes, inhibit histamine release, and inhibit the dilation of the blood vessels and subsequent swelling.

While bioflavonoids occur in the same foods mentioned above for vitamin C, they are also present in rose hips, plums, cherries, blackcurrants, eggplant, squash, parsley, and red wine. Vitamin supplements that contain both vitamin C and bioflavonoids are very easy to find, and the dosage recommendation is still based on a vitamin C content of 500 mg taken morning and night.

Two more very strong antioxidants are *Pycnogenol* and grape seed extract, which are chemically the same but come from different sources. Pycnogenol, a registered trademark, is extracted from the bark of maritime pine trees, whereas grape seed extract (obviously) comes from grape seeds. Since it's much easier to gain access to grape seeds, a waste product of the wine industry, than it is to strip the bark off trees, grape seed extract is less expensive.

It's estimated that grape seed extract is an antioxidant **twenty times** more powerful than vitamin C (this doesn't mean that you still don't need the vitamin C for connective tissue repair, protection against infection, and support of the adrenal glands: you should take both). An effective dosage of grape seed extract is 50 mg three times a day.

Other antioxidants include beta-carotene, vitamin E, and selenium.

However, the goal of this book is not to see how many pills you can stuff into your body. These other antioxidants can be obtained by simply taking a good-quality multiple vitamin, which I will discuss shortly.

The Importance of Pure water

It's very important to note that if you're going to take antioxidants, then you must drink water throughout the day to flush the free radicals out of your body. Of course, you should be drinking water throughout the day anyway, but it becomes especially important in this case so that you don't have all these toxins being released with no way out of your body.

The quality of the water that you're drinking is also very important. I personally believe that everyone needs to buy a water filter for his or her home. They come in many forms, from the inexpensive to the space age varieties that filter every faucet in the house. Even if you can't afford a thousand-dollar system, there are simple filtration devices that require nothing more than putting water into a container that has a filter in it.

I don't think it's a good idea to trust our public water systems because of all the chemicals in the ground that are leaching into the water supplies. Some brands of bottled water can be suspect, as the quality varies so much, and some studies have found companies putting regular tap water into the bottles (unlike in Europe, US bottled water standards are close to nonexistent). The more expensive brands of bottled water probably live up to their claims of purity, but the cost would make drinking them on a daily basis prohibitive, and they are more appropriate for those times when you're away from home.

While distilled water is very pure and sounds like a good solution to treated and/or polluted water, there's a problem with its total lack of mineral content. Part of the value of drinking water is that it's a source of minerals. Nature abhors a vacuum, and unless your diet is exceptionally high in minerals, the distilled water is going to dilute the mineral concentration in your body. So, in the long run, it's best to buy some form of water filtration system for your home, and if you're traveling or away from home, buy a good-quality bottled water.

Organic Produce and Multiple Vitamins

I would advise you to always buy organic produce whenever possible because the nutritional value is higher and you will be putting fewer toxins into your body. It doesn't make sense to consume produce that's been sprayed with all kinds of chemicals and then take antioxidant pills to try to get the chemicals out of your body.

There used to be some debate, given the way food is grown and produced these days, as to whether you can really get all the essential nutrients from your diet. Recently, however, the American Medical Association (AMA), which up until now has generally scoffed at vitamins and nutritional therapies, put an end to this debate when it issued an advisory recommending that everyone should take a multiple vitamin on a daily basis. A good approach is to find a really good-quality multiple vitamin and mineral supplement in a health food or vitamin store and take it every day. While it's still essential that you have a well-balanced diet, this should fill in any nutritional gaps that might exist.

By adopting a commonsense approach to the foods you choose to eat, understanding your relationship with food, and making a commitment to treat your body with the respect it deserves, you'll lose weight (if you need to) and feel so much better by having the proper fuel your body requires to function at its optimal level.

NO WONDER YOU FEEL LIKE CRAP!

PSYCHOLOGICAL STRESS

"It's all in your mind, you know." — George Harrison

Although the focus of this book is primarily on the relationship between the physiological stressors of pain, intestinal tract and systemic inflammation, and unbalanced cortisol levels, it's important that we discuss the role of psychological stress as well. Acute psychological stress will raise cortisol levels just as much as physical pain and inflammation and, if it becomes chronic, it can eventually lead to adrenal gland burnout and cortisol depletion.

Of equal importance is the fact that, for some people, chronic psychological stress can cause intestinal tract irritation and inflammation, and thus perpetuate the physiological stress scenarios discussed in the previous chapter. Keeping in mind that each person's body can respond to stress differently, elevated cortisol levels in some people will inhibit the normal tissue repair necessary for the digestive tract to counterbalance the daily onslaught of caustic acids the body produces to digest food. The progressive inflammation caused by the acids will then further raise the cortisol levels, and we're back to the vicious cycle of interplay between the two types of stress: physiological and psychological.

For most people, "I'm so stressed out!" is the catch phrase that defines their lives. According to people's daily conversations, the prevalence of stress in their lives appears to have reached epidemic proportions. It comes from your job, your boss, your spouse or significant other, your kids, your parents, your siblings, your computer, your television, your newspaper, other drivers, and the guy in the nine items-or-less / cash-only express checkout line at the grocery store with fifteen items and his checkbook. It seems everyone is stressed out about something these days, and stress is a major focal point in many a discussion.

The Subjective Perception of Stress

The single most intriguing aspect of psychological stress is that it's almost completely subjective. I think most people would initially disagree with this because we all harbor the illusion that our reactions to our stressors are "normal" and "correct," e.g., the old "who wouldn't be angry/mad/upset?" in response to a certain set of circumstances. There's also a list of the top ten stressors considered to be universal, such as the death of a loved one, the loss of employment, divorce, and so on.

However, consider the divorce in which one person doesn't want the dissolution of the marriage and will be left brokenhearted and burdened with the role of single parent, while the other person will be embarking on a romantic adventure with a new partner; or maybe the spouse who, left behind to be the single parent, is thrilled to see the abusive lout finally leave.

Another example of the subjectivity of the stress response would be the death of a loved one, the obvious response to which would be intense grief. However, if the circumstances of the loved one's death involved horrible, prolonged suffering from the ravages of cancer, then the emotional response might be one of relief that the person's pain has ended, in which case the grief might be a good deal less. Allowing for different cultural perspectives, some societies view death as a joyous occasion on which the loved one is passing on to a far better place, and so there is no need to mourn his or her departure. It's all a matter of what you believe to be true.

The famous philosopher J. Krishnamurti would often take questions from audiences following his lectures. His most common response to all of these very sincere questions, which were usually concerned with the disharmony among people, how peace could be found, the meaning of life, or the nature of love, was "Why do you think that?" This response would usually cause the person asking the question to try to rephrase it, as if Krishnamurti didn't understand the original one. But after hearing it a second time, Krishnamurti would simply ask again, "Why do you think that?" What he was doing was challenging the rules and beliefs about life and the thinking process that led his listeners to their assumptions and conclusions regarding the human condition. He was asking them to look inside their minds, to follow the constructs that, to them, seemed to form their own brand of "logical, rational thought," and to see where that idea really came from. Krishnamurti had a great awareness and understanding of the subjectivity of human thought and behavior, as well as of the problems it can cause.

Taking Control of What You Think and Feel

How we respond to any given psychological stress is entirely up to us, which by itself is a huge problem. It takes an enormous degree of character to choose to be responsible for all that occurs in your life and to realize that even if you can't control all of the events, you **can** control how you respond and feel about it.

If you decide that no one or nothing can make you feel anything other than what you choose, then you're in possession of great personal power. But it also means you'll have to develop the habit of paying attention to what you're thinking and the why of it. It's easier to blame other people or circumstances for your anger, disappointment, sadness, and failures than to make yourself responsible. It's more tempting to believe something your parents, teachers, or friends told you about how to think or feel, or to go with the flow of popular opinion rather than to have to examine the thought process by which you determine what makes you happy or angry. But like it or not, you're the one who chooses your responses, either actively or passively; and the more you accept that fact, the more control you will have over what you perceive to be stressful.

There's an old saying that goes, "opinions are like assholes—everybody's got one." While the latter serve a useful function, the former often do not. Think for a bit about your day and the internal dialogue you've had with yourself. You know, that wonderful little voice inside your head that either makes you take note of what a beautiful day it is or else whines and moans endlessly about other people's lifestyles, clothing, driving skills, behavior, and on and on. A great question to ask yourself at times when you're on a negative roll is, "Why do I have to have an opinion about this?" Why indeed. What possible good can come from focusing on a litany of negativity as a response to your environment and the people who inhabit it?

People often get trapped in a negative thinking mode. I think part of the problem is that it's fundamental to existence to regard everything we encounter through a survivalist lens, asking first, "Does this present any danger to me?" It is, in fact, how our sensory nervous system works and how we perceive stress. All our sensory information, be it sight, sound, taste, smell, or touch, is first perceived by the limbic system in our brains, which is where our survivalist stress center originates. It's the job of the limbic system to assess the stimulus, decide if it presents a danger to the body, and then initiate the appropriate reaction. If you touch something that's too hot, your limbic system will cause your muscles to contract and move you away from the heat. The limbic system is always evaluating everything that is happening, like a watchful guard dog.

The problem here is that when there isn't much to guard against, when you're safe from harm and on autopilot, your brain just can't be still. We create a lot of mental dialogue and chatter over nothing because we haven't learned how to allow our minds to be still, and because the limbic system is attuned to watching out for negative, dangerous events. We let that little voice inside run rampant as it engages in endless, and mostly useless, monologues in which we just seem to need to have one opinion after another. I think many people learn to look for the negative rather than to focus on the positive, thinking they're doing themselves a favor in a Boy Scout-like effort to "be prepared." A recent research study reports that even in times of prosperity and safety, people still worry a lot and suffer anxiety concerning their future. It's this kind of thought process that gives life to Murphy's Law: the expectation that whatever can go wrong will go wrong.

A better approach to dealing with this mental dialogue is first to be aware of it on a conscious level and not just let it run off on its own, and then to be less judgmental about every little thing. This can be very liberating and at times funny when you catch yourself wasting your time and energy wondering why in the world that teenager's pants are hanging down so low (answer: he's practicing to be a future plumber), or any number of silly things we choose to have an opinion about and clog up our brains with on a daily basis.

This approach of asking yourself why you have to have an opinion about everything gives you an immediately empowering example of how you can actively **choose** your responses instead of allowing your mind to jabber away. Another benefit you'll derive is a sense of less pressure on yourself. This is because judgment implies standards (your own in this case) that you're using to measure yourself against other people. As the Bible says, "Judge not, lest ye be judged." By not being so consumed with comparing yourself to everyone else, you can be more relaxed and accepting of yourself and maintain an attitude of, "live and let live."

Psychological Factors of Stress

In his extraordinary book, *Why Zebras Don't Get Ulcers*, Dr. Robert Sapolsky discusses numerous research studies on the psychological factors of stress. What appear to be the two most important components in the response to this type of stress are **control** and **predictability**.

The amount of control and predictability a human or research animal has, or even perceives it has, greatly determines what effect the stress will have on him or her. In studies, a rat that has some means of controlling the frequency of electric shocks will get fewer ulcers than a rat that has no control. Similarly, a rat that's warned when the shocks will occur will have a less intense stress response than that of the rat given no warning. At some point, if it's shocked frequently enough, the rat will perceive the shock as a predictable stressor and again will have a weaker stress response. A rat that's been trained to use a lever to avoid shocks will have a massive stress response if the lever is taken away; and the stress response will weaken if the lever is returned, even if it's disconnected and doesn't actually prevent the shock from occurring. Just believing that it has some means of control helps the rat reduce its stress levels.

The negative effects of stress and the issue of control apply equally to humans. A recent four-year study conducted by the Harvard Center for Society and Health assessed the effects of job stress on 21,000 women. The study found that a stressful job can cause as much wear and tear on the body as smoking, and that the women in the study who experienced the most job strain also experienced the most health problems. These women were at greater risk for hypertension or high blood pressure as well as for an increased general rate of illness; some even had difficulty walking, climbing stairs, or carrying out their daily activities. This correlates well with my initial assertion that unbalanced levels of cortisol can lead to high blood pressure, immune system dysfunction, and fatigue. What this study also found was that the women who had some control over their schedules and duties were less affected by the stress of their jobs.

It would seem logical that we all want some level of control over the things that occur in our lives and some degree of predictability of events. The problem again comes back to just how much responsibility we want to assume in making our lives as stress-free as possible.

The often incongruous opinions and judgments that make up our thoughts and actions get us into all kinds of trouble. When I was a freshman in college, I had a History professor who began and ended every class with the statement "It's not what **is** that counts, it's what people **think** that counts." Throughout the entire History course he'd prove this point over and over again by illustrating how wars were waged and people slaughtered wholesale on the basis of a belief or a perception of what was "real." How we decide what is stressful to us goes right back to our own perception of what's happening to us, and how that perception coincides with our opinions and judgments.

The best technique I know of for dealing with psychological

stress is to take control and examine your thought process.

Sit yourself down with paper and pen and write down exactly what it is you feel stressed about, then write down **why** you feel stressed about it. In most cases, what will ultimately come to the surface is either a discrepancy between your opinions and judgments about how your life should be and your perceptions of how it is, or a discrepancy between your opinions and judgments and those of someone else; in both cases, stress is the end result of your reaction to the discrepancy.

This would then be a good time to really look at your opinions and judgments and see just exactly where they came from and how much conscious effort went into making them. Do they really make sense and are they reasonable, or are they just a bundle of immature wishes and desires thrown together?

This is a process that can take some time, so don't expect to sit down and get your life and all its stresses worked out in twenty minutes. It also requires some insight and honesty. It can provoke many emotions and at times can even be a little painful because people don't like to admit that they—or what they're thinking—are wrong. But if your opinions and judgments about life are burning up your adrenal glands, then it's better to come to terms with them now before they give you a heart attack or an ulcer.

A compulsive need to be "right" in one's opinions or judgments can cause an enormous amount of pain, both emotional and physical. In my thirty-four years of clinical practice, I've observed numerous cases in which the primary cause of a patient's physical pain was due to an opinion, and the pain was absolutely necessary in order to make that opinion "right." One example would be that of an employee who harbored the unfounded belief that his employer was mean, overbearing, and determined to work people to death, and who consequently developed a pain syndrome that "proved" the destructive intentions of the employer. No amount of treatment would relieve this person's pain, because if the pain was resolved and he was still working for the same employer, then his opinion about his employer would turn out to be "wrong," and that would have been completely unacceptable.

Richard Weinstein, D.C.

Our Opinions and Judgments

Our opinions and judgments in the game of life are actually not hard to understand; they begin as exercises in conditioned response administered by our parents, siblings, schoolmates, teachers, the media, and so on.

When we're very young we learn these rules through trial and error, since our reasoning skills are not yet very well developed. It's impossible for an infant to reason that throwing a bowl of baby food across the room is inappropriate because of the mess it'll make and the extra work this will bring to its parent's already hectic day. So the unreasoning kid will launch the bowl with much glee, only to find its future in aerodynamic research stunted by some immediate form of reprimand or punishment. At this point in its early life, this child does not have a thought-out strategy for managing its response to this stressful experience, and will probably start crying.

As we get older, we experience a lot more of this cause-and-effect business; but with help from our reasoning minds, minds that can foresee the consequences of causing a big mess, we avoid taking the action. So far so good—except that the people who are helping us form our opinions may have some very irrational opinions of their own that they're passing on. Unfortunately, there's nothing that can be done about this, although I personally favor the dog-child rule: before you're allowed to have a kid, you have to get a dog. If you can successfully train the dog, then you get to have a kid. Nevertheless, as we get older, we continue to acquire our opinions and judgments through our experiences and interactions with all manner of people and stimuli, including television.

At some point I think all of us arrive at a place where we begin to question what's going on in our heads (parents know this as adolescence), and we make an effort to determine if what we have been taught to think and feel is valid. But just how committed we are to evaluate this in depth and on an ongoing basis will greatly affect our ability to manage our emotions, behavior, and responses to stress. If you're being conditioned by a bad parent or teacher to believe that you're stupid, lazy, worthless, and won't amount to anything of value, you're doomed—unless you take it upon yourself to question and challenge these assumptions. People who survive adverse childhood conditions of abuse, poverty, and violence do so by making their own evaluations of these situations and adopting rules and beliefs that defy their circumstances.

I'm not suggesting a micromanagement approach to evaluating every thought or feeling you have, because that will lead to obsessive-compulsive behavior, and then you'll be plenty stressed out. What would be more appropriate would be to do an initial checkup on yourself, looking at the more significant opinions and judgments you have now, and to see if they make sense and enhance your life.

For example, harboring an opinion/judgment that for me to be happy I absolutely must be a multimillionaire living in Tahiti while dating members of the Swedish womens' volleyball team is probably not going to make for a stress-free existence. On the other hand, if I construct my life around opinions and judgments that enable me to be a positive influence on other people's lives, making every day count, having goals to achieve, and counting my blessings, then it's going to be a lot easier to be content at the end of each day. If I insist on having opinions that are immature, unrealistic, or incongruous, then I'm setting myself up for failure and disappointment.

Being in Charge of Your Life

Most people spend more time planning their annual two-week vacation than they do planning the rest of their lives. They wake up and basically let the day happen to them rather than start out with a proactive concept of what they want the day to be like, what they want to accomplish, and what kind of relationship they want to have with the people they will encounter.

Every day people drag themselves off to work with no better chance of things going consistently well than if they were to get in a boat with no compass and push off the dock in the hope they'll land in Tahiti. Since Dr. Sapolsky's research clearly shows that the two major components of psychological stress are control and predictability, it makes a great deal of sense to begin each day by having at least a concept or "prediction" of what you wish to have happen. Obviously not everything will go as planned, but at least you're starting out with some sense of control, and as long as you don't have a rule that says everything must go as planned or you'll shoot yourself, you'll probably feel less stressed out. Remember that the rat that believes it has control even if the lever that would prevent the shock doesn't work still has a less intense response to stress. So how hard would it be to take a few minutes at the beginning of each day to think about what kind of day you wish to have in order to gain a sense of control over your life? Or to decide that nothing is going to make you angry or upset and that **you**— not someone else—will choose how you feel? Or that you don't have to have an opinion about every little thing you see or hear?

Another example of taking control is to look at your attitude when you arrive home from work each day. Do you take a moment to compose yourself and actively think about what kind of relationship you want to have with your spouse, kids, or whomever, or do you just leap out of the car, bound through the door, and see what happens next? How much control and predictability is involved in that? Or do you expect to be treated a certain way because you worked hard today, without considering that the other people in your life have their own expectations, and that these might not be totally compatible with yours?

Again, the more you become aware of how and what you're thinking and the more you're consciously directing your life, the less stress you'll encounter.

Taking Action

With any technique designed to help manage psychological stress, success depends on action; this means that you can read about stress reduction all day long and understand the concept very well, but until you actually **do** something to change your stress response, nothing is really going to change. This is where some stress-management techniques run into trouble: because they're too time-consuming, they end up as just another stressor.

The activities I'm recommending are easy and don't take much time; in fact, they've been designed to be done in small increments to ensure success.

The following activities don't have to be done in any particular order, so just start with the ones that seem the easiest and most comfortable to do, but plan on doing all of them at some point—above all, don't quit. Since it's easier to learn a new habit when it's linked with something you're already doing on a daily basis, here's a list of actions you can take based on just this approach.

- Give yourself five extra minutes before you get out of bed in the morning to reflect on what kind of day you want to have; what objectives you want to achieve; what kinds of emotions you want to experience. If you were a movie director going to the set to film today's scene of *Your Life*, what would the movie look like at the end of the day's shooting?

- When you're taking your shower or bath, don't let your mind get filled up with a bunch of gibberish but be fully present and feel the physical sensation of the hot water, the smell of the soap, and the massaging of the shampoo in your hair. Then take a moment to realize how lucky you are to have indoor plumbing, hot water, and a working bathroom, which hundreds of millions of people throughout the world do not.

- Every time before you eat, take fifteen seconds (or longer if you wish) to be grateful for actually having something to eat, and remember that not everyone in this world is so fortunate.

- If you're in a relationship with a "significant other", find a reason or an opportunity every day to tell that person that you love him or her. Life is short, and you don't want to regret missing any chance to bring happiness into your lover's life.

- Whether or not you're romantically involved with someone, you're still in a relationship with the world around you. On your way to and from work or while running errands, turn down the mental noise in your head and turn up your senses, paying attention to the sights and sounds around you. Noticing the incredible natural beauty of the world you live in also has the reciprocal effect of turning down that mental noise, so that the more aware you are, the less stressed out you'll be.

- In addition to the relationship you may have with a lover or with the physical world in which you exist, there's your relationship and interdependence with a myriad of people who directly impact your life and make it "work." I very much enjoy being a doctor and love my job, but I'm acutely aware that without my office staff, the grocery clerk, my waste-disposal service, my car mechanic, and a whole host of other people and the services they provide for me, my life would be far more difficult. You come into contact with these people on a daily basis. Be appreciative of all of the people who affect your life and show them your appreciation.

- Beyond all of these external relationships is the one you have with yourself. Each day find a reason to tell yourself that you love **you**—because of a good deed you've done, because you accomplished what you set out to do, or simply because you found some enjoyment in that particular day. Taking a few minutes before going to sleep to reflect upon your day and how you lived it is a good way to end your day.

- Get a good old-fashioned paper calendar that has each month on a separate page. At the beginning of each month, on a separate piece of paper, write down a list of five things you're currently worried about. Then take that list and tape it to the next month's page. At the end of the month when you turn to the next month's page and find your list, see how important those worries were—or if they even still exist, since you've quite possibly come up with a whole new list of worries! This is a good way to gain some perspective on what we **think** is stressful and on just how transitory these worries can be. Of course, if you're dealing with your own serious illness or that of a loved one, an extended period of unemployment, or your burned-down house, then the stress may certainly extend into the next month; but, by and large, you'll come to realize that many of the things you worried about weren't worth the bother in the first place.

Hormone Imbalance and Rational Thinking

There's no doubt that having a clearer understanding of what your opinions and judgments really are, seeing how they impact your life on a daily basis, deciding to take charge of your life, and then implementing a positive plan of action that enables you to manage stress more effectively by giving you a greater sense of control and predictability, will enhance the quality of your life. Learning to handle psychological stress better is certainly important, because not doing so is going to result in elevated levels of cortisol and a myriad of related physical problems.

However, this is a good place to come to terms with the fact that if your cortisol levels are already chronically elevated due to physical inflammation, then it's entirely possible that the cortisol imbalance will impede your ability to cope with psychological stress. It's the vicious cycle again.

Numerous researchers have documented the fact that the nerve cells in our brains can be ravaged by elevated levels of cortisol, especially in the hippocampus and amygdale, the two parts of our brain which make perceptual judgments about incoming information. Our ability to make rational sense of our world is dependent on how well these nerve cells work, and elevated levels of cortisol can impair their function.

This is why, if you have the symptoms described in earlier chapters, it's so important to have your cortisol levels tested. It will be very difficult for you to rationally assess the quality of your opinions and judgments, or to do well in any of the other areas of psychological stress management that we've been discussing, if your cortisol levels are impairing the very areas of the brain that you use to make these judgments.

Richard Weinstein, D.C.

THE EMOTIONAL COMPONENT OF ILLNESS

A Tricky Roadblock on the Way to Regaining Good Health

Congratulations! You've conquered your pain syndrome, repaired your intestinal lining, and your cortisol/DHEA ratios are normal.

But what's that you say? You still don't feel too spunky?

If that's the case, it's now time to come full circle from the discussion of psychological stress in Chapter 9 to the emotional component of illness. Not everyone who has a pain syndrome or a chronic illness will necessarily have this emotional component, and of those who do, some cases may be much more complicated than others.

It's easy to understand why people who suffer a lot of pain that limits their lifestyle and interrupts their sleep might be depressed or irritable. And if, in addition to a pain-inducing structural disorder, they also suffer from the chemical component of leaky gut syndrome and cortisol imbalances, then it's all that much easier to understand why they don't feel well emotionally.

For many people, all it takes is the resolution of their structural and chemical problems to restore them physically and mentally to their usual selves. Unfortunately, some people get their physical problems resolved but continue to not thrive. Either their problems transform into some new complaint, or the old ones have a nasty way of recurring. In these cases, the emotional component of illness must be explored.

NO WONDER YOU FEEL LIKE CRAP!

The Three Factors of the Emotional Component

In my experience treating patients, there are usually three factors at play in the emotional arena. The first has to do with something known as *learned helplessness*; the second concerns *control-coping skills*; and the last factor has to do with *subconscious conditioned-response triggers*. These factors can occur separately or in combination.

Learned Helplessness

Learned helplessness is a term used to describe an animal that's been conditioned in such a way that it can no longer cope appropriately with even the most mundane tasks in its life.

In laboratory experiments two groups of rats were exposed to huge amounts of stress, and then tested for how a degree of control and predictability would affect the rats response to the stress.

The first group of rats was trained in what is known as an active-avoidance task. This was accomplished by putting a rat in a cage where half the floor would transmit an electrical shock and in which, prior to giving the shock, the rat would be given a signal indicating which side of the floor would become electrified. Once it had learned the signal, the rat would reliably move to the side of the cage that would not transmit the shock. These rats did not show any increased signs of stress because they'd learned how to control their situation.

The second group of rats was exposed to frequent electrical shocks and noise over a long period of time with no warning, no ability to control the stimuli, and no sense of predictability as to when they would occur. These rats exhibited many of the same characteristics seen in human depression: elevated cortisol levels, disturbed sleep cycles, and a loss of motivation.

When this second group was placed in the same environment as the first group of rats, where signals and warnings were given before the shocks, they were unable to learn the active-avoidance task. Even attempts to reward the rats beyond enabling them to avoid the shocks, such as giving them food or sex, failed to change their behavior. It seems that once the rats were conditioned into learned helplessness, embracing the perception that there was nothing they could do to change or improve their situation, they were permanently damaged in their ability to cope **even when the dynamics of their situation changed.**

Learned helplessness has been demonstrated in studies using dogs, cats, birds, and humans. There are frightening and insidious implications in how easily some human beings can be conditioned into learned helplessness. Going back to one of the most basic premises of this book, each individual responds differently to stress, which is a very fortunate thing. Unfortunately, there are studies on underprivileged children that show that their overall inability to read was a result of their being conditioned to believe that they were intellectually incapable of the task.

Let's take a look at how learned helplessness can become a factor in a pain syndrome or chronic illness.

You'll recall that Dr. Robert Sapolsky, the Stanford University stress researcher, states that the two greatest psychological stressors are the lack of control and lack of predictability. So there you are, with a chronic pain syndrome, leaky gut, systemic inflammation, and you feel as if your body is sabotaging you. Sometimes you hurt, sometimes you don't; the pain wanders around, and the degree of pain varies from tolerable to intolerable. Some nights you sleep, and some nights you're wide awake staring at the ceiling. Some days you're tense and irritable, and other days you're so lethargic you can barely move. You don't understand what in the world is wrong with you, and your loved ones are beginning to wonder about you as well. It seems you have no control over how you're going to feel from one day to the next, nor can you predict which activities you may or may not engage in. This is when the emotional stress adds to the stress you already have from physical pain and gastrointestinal inflammation, and when your adrenal glands' ability to manage the stress is progressively declining.

Now, logic would suggest that after resolving the structural pain syndrome and the chemical cortisol imbalance, your emotional life would just go back to normal. But as we've seen with the experiments on learned helplessness, that's not always the case. For some people who have experienced chronic or repetitive episodes of pain or long-term cortisol imbalances, learned helplessness becomes part of their personality. The prolonged pain and/or cortisol imbalance changes both their external perception of the world around them and their internal perception of their ability to cope with that world. They become fearful of activity because they think it might produce pain, and they don't allow themselves to do things that were once a source of fun. They no longer go skiing or dancing, and they avoid long trips because they're afraid these activities will cause a recurrence of pain.

These people become socially withdrawn because they're so used to being anxious, depressed, or both, that they don't feel very comfortable around other people. They've learned not to trust their bodies and are waiting for the next bad thing to happen, as it always has in the past. Even when they're not in any pain and there's no intestinal inflammation causing an elevation of cortisol, they continue to sleep poorly because they go to bed worrying if it'll be a good night or a bad night, and the worrying raises cortisol levels to the point where they cause insomnia.

This brings us to the mind/body research study being done at the University of Iowa, where researchers using brain scans measure blood flow to different parts of the brain while the test subjects think of specific emotions. What this study revealed is that certain emotions will influence neurological activity in parts of the brain that are also associated with muscle and organ function. So what may be happening in learned helplessness with regard to illness is a case of self-fulfilling prophecy, meaning that the constant worry or expectation of bad things occurring causes a negative neurological stimulus in the part of the brain that will actually **cause** these bad things to happen. This just reaffirms the helplessness, and the cycle continues.

Control–Coping Skills

The second factor in the emotional component of illness is the control-coping skill, which is a kind of bizarre twist on learned helplessness. It involves using the illness to regain control and predictability over one's life. In most cases, I think this starts out innocently enough as a fair response to being ill or in pain, but over time it takes on a life of its own and grows from being subconscious to subtly intentional.

This factor has its origin in childhood, when we discover that we can stay home from school and get lots of attention if we become ill. That works well until one day we realize that we forgot to do a book report or study for a test, and we fake being sick to get out of going to school. Since our parents surely tried this trick on their parents, they're not so easily fooled, and you end up suffering the double whammy of having to go to school unprepared along with the punishment you will receive when you get home for trying to pull such a stunt. This is usually enough to teach you to not make a career out of being "sick."

However, some people learn a very different lesson about being ill. What they learn is that because they're ill, the people around them are sympathetic and give them more attention. They also can't be expected to clean the house, do the dishes, mow the lawn, or seek gainful employment. Should the people around them begin to complain about their prolonged illness, they are only going to get sicker from the additional stress, and God knows we wouldn't want **that** to happen!. So the person who's ill now gets to decide if and when certain activities take place, like going on trips or going to a movie (and which movie it will be, lest he has to sit too long or watch something that might upset him), or if there might be sex that night, and in just what position… And the list goes on and on.

This is not to say that these people don't have some or all of the physical problems I've previously discussed, such as pain syndromes, intestinal tract and/or systemic inflammation, and cortisol imbalances. It's just that they've learned to use their illnesses to control virtually every aspect of their lives either consciously or subconsciously. The world revolves around them, and all decisions regarding family, friends, employment, and activities, are regulated by how they feel.

To make matters worse, look at what they stand to lose should they ever get well: their entire lives will change in ways they may perceive as not particularly desirable. The idea of having to return to being a regular person whose needs don't supersede anyone else's after months or—more typically—years of being in control and being relieved of many responsibilities, can be frightening. The concept of going back to work, being socially engaged, and having additional responsibilities after years of dealing with pain and stress-related disorders can seem overwhelming and—of course—very stressful. So while their physical conditions might improve over time, they never really get well and instead linger at some plateau that enables them to remain in control.

One aspect of control-coping skill and how it relates to learned helplessness is that these people decide that certain activities are the cause of their problems and, therefore, must be avoided forever. For example, if you're suffering from lower back pain, which is frequently caused by activities that require bending forward, you might perceive vacuuming the carpet as a very risky task. Even if you recover from the back pain, you might decide that you must never vacuum again because you consider it a causative factor. The fact that you can vacuum a rug without bending forward by just pushing the upright vacuum cleaner while standing up straight has never occurred to you. But, most important, with your control-coping skill you've found a way to get someone else to do the vacuuming.

As the person gains more control, they can arrive at the conclusion that they pretty much can't do **anything** without getting into trouble, so they decide that it's better to do nothing and to have other people perform these physical tasks. A more appropriate response would be to learn to do these activities using proper bending and lifting techniques (always bend from the knees, not from the waist) and to consult a physical therapist or personal trainer in order to get into better physical shape.

All this, however, brings us back to the fear or dread of the trappings of a "normal" life and the perceived stress inherent in being well and not having any valid reasons for being excused from the everyday responsibilities that affect most people.

When I encounter this behavior in patients, I find it important not to criticize the person but to make them aware of it. This is not hypochondria or a psychological disorder; this is a coping skill that they've learned in the face of chronic pain and hormonal imbalance. In the example I gave earlier about hormones overriding rational thought (should you eat that candy bar?), you'll recall that the hormonally-induced craving always wins; this is the same thing. Even though patients may be responding well to treatment, the fear they associate with their condition and activity can still cause an elevation of cortisol, which keeps them going around in circles. So while the logical part of their brains rationally concludes that being healthy is a desirable thing, the hormonal chemicals in their brains induce a fear that is hard to overcome.

By making patients aware of this syndrome, they can begin to realize more clearly what their fears are and how they may be sabotaging their efforts to get well. I find it useful to have them go home and write down five positive and five negative changes that would occur in their lives if they were completely healthy. As you might imagine, some patients get defensive and declare that there are no negative aspects to their getting well; but when I ask them when was the last time they cleaned the house, mowed the lawn, raked the leaves, took out the garbage, washed the car, and so on, they get the idea.

I also challenge them to re-evaluate why they think that being healthy will mean that they have to change their lives in a way they associate with stress. After all, if they haven't been doing these tasks for months or years, why do they assume they'll have to do them now? Obviously these responsibilities are being managed in some other way, and perhaps there's no reason for them to feel that an overwhelming wave of new obligations will come crashing down on them simply because they're no longer physically impaired.

It's also very important to remind them that just because they've had problems in the past, it doesn't mean they're destined to have them in the future. By achieving success in a good treatment program, by learning the correct biomechanics of how to use their bodies to avoid re-injury, and by having their hormonal imbalances resolved, they can move on with their lives. They will have gained the knowledge of what went wrong and know that not only can it be corrected, it also can be prevented from recurring. Knowledge is a powerful tool.

Subconscious Conditioned-Response Triggers

This brings us to the third factor in the emotional component of getting well: subconscious conditioned-response triggers.

Even after resolving their pain syndromes and hormonal imbalances, and armed with the strategies for dealing successfully with their health, sometimes patients can't align themselves with their thoughts and emotions. They understand their health issues intellectually, but they simply can't get past their conditioned responses. These subconscious triggers often play a significant role in the learned helplessness and control-coping skills components.

As it pertains to learned helplessness, patients who have successfully recovered from their pain syndromes and/or cortisol imbalances understand intellectually that they should be able to lift objects or to garden without ending up in pain, or be able to sleep or encounter social situations without unnecessary anxieties. However, they're not "emotionally congruent," and the mere sight of a wheelbarrow or the thought of being involved in a situation that used to cause pain or anxiety triggers a fear response that prevents them from properly adapting to the situation.

The control/coping skills component is equally vulnerable to subconscious triggers. While people who are using a physical disorder as a means of controlling their environment are busy assuring themselves and those around them that they really want to get well, they remain emotionally incongruent with the concept of being well and losing control.

A good example of this is provided by Ivan Pavlov and his hallmark research with dogs and conditioned responses. By consistently ringing a bell before feeding the dogs, Pavlov conditioned the dogs to associate food with the bell and to salivate when they heard the bell. Even when he stopped feeding them after ringing the bell, the dogs continued to salivate when the bell rang.

The same process occurs in the human model, where you know intellectually that there's no reason to metaphorically "salivate" just because you "hear the bell," but your conditioning is so strong that **you do it anyway**. For human beings, it doesn't require repetitive reinforcement to anchor the conditioning; often the conditioning is the result of a single emotionally charged moment.

The problem is, during a highly charged emotional event, the perception of what's happening and the meaning that the brain attaches to it may not be completely rooted in reality. Nevertheless, these events get stored in our memory banks and can be triggered by other sensory stimuli that might have been circumstantially present when the original event occurred.

Events make a biochemical impression on the brain, specifically in the hippocampus, which, as previously discussed, deals with short-term memory. To file experiences away permanently, the hippocampus shunts the elements of the experience—the sounds, smells, sights—through a network of nerve cells to different areas of the brain. The proper stimulus (say, a whiff of perfume or a glimpse of a familiar place) trips the relay, firing the neurons and bringing a past event into consciousness.

A great way to test this is to turn on the radio to what would be an "oldies" station relative to your age group and see how different songs trigger memories of where you were at that time, the friends you had, and even of a particular girlfriend or boyfriend. Some songs will seem like the theme of an entire summer or will remind you of your first kiss or the times you drove around with your friends with hardly a care in the world. Or pull out that shoe box of pictures collecting dust under your bed and see how looking at them brings up memories of the people and events that were taking place when the pictures were snapped. After all, isn't that the whole purpose of taking pictures in the first place?

The downside of this is that a stimulus can also trigger an unconscious response of an emotionally negative experience, which then neurologically inhibits the normal function of an organ or muscle group (referring back to the research at the University of Iowa that shows the association of emotions linked to the parts of the brain that relate to specific organs and muscles).

Tragically, childhood victims of physical or sexual abuse are prone to these responses. The San Francisco Spine Institute, which deals with patients with complicated and serious spinal disorders, has found that there's a higher incidence of chronic back pain in people who have suffered such childhood abuse. One possible reason for this may be the conditioned response of tightening the lower back muscles to arch the back in an attempt to elude an attack.

But what happens when these people, as adults, encounter a sensory stimulus that unconsciously triggers a memory of an attack? Suppose they go to the grocery store and encounter a perfume or cologne that smells like that of their attacker; just then, as they bend to put their groceries in the car, their back goes into a spasm? In the course of their lifetime they may have put hundreds of bags of groceries into their vehicle with no problem, but in this instance their back muscles are emotionally prompted into such a state of tension that just a small physical movement triggers a complete spasm.

Emotional Stress and Neck and Lower Back Pain

There appears to be a high correlation between stress and neck/lower back pain. And although there's definitive research that shows that all primates will tense their trapezius muscles (those great big muscles that attach the neck to the shoulders and that you love to have massaged) when stressed or angered, no one knows why. After thirty-four years of practice and thinking about this, my clinical hunch is that there's a neurological connection between the nerves of the neck and lower back and the adrenal glands.

There's a group of nerves that emerges from the vertebrae of the neck, called the *brachial plexus*, which comprises the entire nerve supply of the upper limbs. Similarly, the group of nerves exiting the vertebrae of the lower back forms the *lumbosacral plexus*, which furnishes the entire nerve supply to the lower limbs. The human response to stress is often referred to as the fight-or-flight syndrome, which implies that you're going to resolve a physically threatening situation by using either your arm muscles for fighting or your leg muscles for fleeing to safety, or some combination of both. Since the adrenal glands orchestrate this response, it's highly probable that cortisol stimulates the function of these neurological plexuses to carry out the muscular functions necessary to survive the stress.

This response to stress, and the firing of these neurological plexuses, are great if you're wrestling an alligator or being chased by a mountain lion. But if the stress is psychological or the cortisol level is elevated by inflammation, and the arm and leg muscles are not involved in fighting or fleeing, then activating the nerve plexuses of the neck and lower back is probably a prescription for pain and nothing more. It's very common for people to say that they hold their stress in their neck and upper back muscles (the trapezius muscles), and the statement is neurologically correct. We also seem to know intuitively that stress affects these areas, as we frequently refer to stressful situations or people as being a pain in the neck or a pain in the ass.

In many of these instances the stress is transitory and the muscles relax, returning to their pre-stress status. However, should the stress be prolonged or related to a highly charged emotional event, then the muscles may remain fixated, restricting the ability of the spinal joints to move normally, and result in joint dysfunction and pain. If the stress response is triggered by an emotional event, then this syndrome can go on forever, and patients may not understand why they keep having problems.

Resolving Conditioned-Response Triggers

Fortunately, there's a treatment technique that addresses these negative emotionally charged conditioned responses that interfere with normal physical function, and it's called *Neuro-Emotional Technique* (NET). This technique, created by Dr. Scott Walker, a chiropractor from Encinitas, California, is based on the current research regarding *neuropeptides*, which are the chemicals that transmit emotions.

Dr. Walker's work embraces the reality that emotional events can get locked into different parts of our bodies, and he terms these events *neuro-emotional complexes* (NECs). Furthermore, he states that not all NECs correspond with actual or historical reality, as they may be the result of perceptual misconceptions, and so he views NECs as the patient's emotional reality. It's this reality that the patient experienced and remembers, proving once again that most of life, and stress, is perceptual.

Neuro-Emotional Technique is a methodology used to normalize negative physical and/or behavioral patterns that have become locked into the body. Just as the researchers from the University of Iowa are seeing the neurological correlation between emotions and organ/muscle function, NET makes these same connections and assists in eliminating these negative patterns.

Dr. Elmer Green, the Mayo Clinic physician who pioneered biofeedback as a treatment for disease, has stated that "every change in the physiological state is accompanied by an appropriate change in the mental/emotional state, conscious or unconscious; and conversely, every change in the mental/emotional state, conscious or unconscious, is accompanied by an appropriate change in the physiological state."

Candace B. Pert, Ph.D., was one of the leading researchers at the National Institutes of Health in a study to find opiate receptors in the brain, which led to the discovery of endorphins (our own naturally-produced pain-relieving chemicals) and the subsequent mapping of the brain's neurotransmitter receptor sites. In her book, *Molecules of Emotion*, she describes in detail the body-mind relationship between the neurotransmitter chemicals of emotions and somatic, or physical, function. She goes on to say: "Most psychologists treat the mind as disembodied, a phenomenon with little or no connection to the physical body. Conversely, physicians treat the body with little or no regard to the mind or the emotions. But the body and mind are not separate, and we cannot treat one without the other. My research has shown me that the body can and must be healed through the mind, and the mind can and must be healed through the body."

Dr. Pert has worked in a research project with Dr. Walker that seeks to develop further applications of the neuro-emotional technique to correct mind/body imbalances.

The Wedding Bell Blues

One example of how emotional stressors can bring about physical pain involves one of my middle-aged male patients who was responding very well to treatment for a chronic lower back pain condition. Although he wasn't supposed to return to my office for a week, he called in for an emergency appointment because of the sudden return of intense pain. When he arrived at my office, the most obvious question to ask was what exactly had happened and when did the pain begin. He stated that he had done no physical activity leading up to the onset of the pain and that he first experienced the pain while seated in a movie theater with his wife.

I performed my usual analysis of his spine, determined which areas needed correction, and proceeded with my chiropractic treatment. My experience, however, told me there was probably more to this than an ergonomically incorrect movie theater seat as the causal factor in his back pain, so I tested him for a neuro-emotional complex.

In this particular case, it turned out that he and his wife had been debating over which movie to see, and although he really didn't want to see the one she'd chosen, they saw it anyway. So there he was, sitting in the movie theater, grumbling all the way through a movie he'd already decided he hated before he even saw it, and the stress caused his back to go into a spasm so that he could barely get up out of his chair by the time the movie was over.

Now, at first glance, this would all seem to be a rather immature response to something as silly as a movie, but there's more.

Further testing revealed that this was just the tip of the iceberg and that the origin of this type of emotional response for him was his wedding, which had taken place thirty-eight years ago! He'd wanted a small, intimate wedding with just close family and friends, but his lovely bride-to-be had insisted on a major extravaganza that included nearly every person she'd ever known in her life. He conceded and let her have her way, and it had been gnawing at him for all the years since. Now, when a similar contentious situation arose, it literally rang his wedding bells and resulted in an emotional charge that affected his body. By using the neuro-emotional technique, we broke the connection between the emotional response and the corresponding physical reaction. After thirty-eight years of carrying around these emotions, it's probable that similar emotional conflicts will arise, but with this technique, the *physical* consequences will not reoccur.

Being "Right" Can Be Very Painful

An example of one of the most tragic and extreme examples of a neuro-emotional complex as the underlying cause of a pain syndrome involved a forty-two-year-old man who had a work-related lifting injury that resulted in unusually severe back pain. The man was originally employed by a state-of-the-art medical supply company that shipped high-tech surgical tools to hospitals, sometimes on immediate notice in order to save someone's life. He was in charge of handling the phone orders and getting the shipments out, a job with a lot of control and, in his perception, power.

Unfortunately, as time went on and the company's competitors developed more advanced surgical tools, business slowed down dramatically, and the company was looking to downsize by getting rid of employees with the most seniority and the highest wages. Because the company's employees were unionized, it was not easy to simply fire people without incurring legal difficulties, so they transferred this guy to the shipping department. In his mind, he went from a powerful white-collar job to a guy in overalls doing manual labor.

The actual event that caused his injury was lifting a five-pound box of surgical gloves. It resulted in intense, debilitating lower back pain that forever changed his life. He was treated by orthopedic specialists, neurologists, and physical therapists. He received cortisone injections in his spine, eventually had two surgeries to try to relieve nerve pressure, and—finding little to no resolution for his pain—was placed on lifetime disability. Thus a big lawsuit followed.

When he came to see me ten years after the initial injury, he was still in considerable pain and unable to sit, stand, or walk comfortably. It was obvious from our first consultation that he blamed his former employer for everything that was wrong with his life, and it occurred to me that there was probably a neuro-emotional complex involved in his pain syndrome.

I don't usually start with the neuro-emotional technique on a patient's first visit, but this guy had been through so much other care for his back pain with such minimal results that I thought it was in his best interest to at least explore this avenue. I explained to him that while there was certainly something structurally wrong with his spine, there might also be a chemical or emotional component that was contributing to his pain. He was pretty much willing to try anything at this point, so after examining him and treating him with spinal manipulation, I tested him for a neuro-emotional complex.

In going through the procedure it became apparent that the emotional content underlying his back pain was anger, and it was quite a revelation to him when he realized that it was his bitter anger at being demoted that was actually causing most of his pain. What became clear to him was that, in his mind, he couldn't get well because if he did, he'd have to go back to a job that he perceived as humiliating and beneath his qualifications. It was emotionally so painful to go back to that job that the emotion subconsciously transformed into physical pain, which made him unable to work. In addition, his physical condition justified—at least in his mind—his blame and hatred for the company, like a bad song playing continuously in his head. This man actually recovered to the point where his pain was so diminished (having two surgeries does tend to permanently alter normal spinal dynamics) that he was able to return to work as a consultant for another company.

The lesson to be learned from this, and it's one that I frequently mention to other patients with similar issues, is that sometimes being "right" can be a very painful experience. Harboring anger, blame, animosity, and resentment in the name of being justified or "right" in one's opinions and beliefs can lead to all kinds of mischief and negative health consequences. To paraphrase Mother Teresa, no matter how large the hurt or anger is, there comes a time when you simply have to let it go and move on with your life. This patient, who had wasted years of his life being angry and in pain, finally ended up doing what he should have done in the first place, which was to leave a job he no longer liked and transfer his talent and expertise to a new employer.

These are cases of patients whose pain syndromes were not resolved by using physical modalities (chiropractic manipulation, physical therapy, massage, surgery) or hormonal/nutritional balancing, because the driving force behind their pain had an emotional component. This is not to imply that every person with a pain syndrome has an emotional basis for it, or that if there is one, it has to be due to some severe emotional trauma; sometimes a persistent pain in the neck is nothing more emotionally charged than having a coworker who's particularly irritating. But if seeing that person five days a week is the cause of your pain, then the neuro-emotional technique is an excellent way to resolve it.

It's very important to note that neuro-emotional technique does not, nor was ever intended to, replace psychiatric care or psychological counseling. But it certainly can be a helpful adjunct in cases where a patient has received such care and in the process has come to an intellectual understanding of his problems but continues to respond negatively to the same old triggers. In such cases Neuro-Emotional Technique can be enormously beneficial.

Richard Weinstein, D.C.

CONCLUSION

We've come full circle in exploring all the components of stress and how to cope with each one of them. Hopefully, you're now able to see stress in a very different light and to realize that it may not be your external circumstances alone that are causing you to feel stressed out, but that, in many instances, it has more to do with your internal structural, chemical, and emotional well-being.

Whether or not this requires seeking appropriate treatment to relieve pain and eliminate the need for NSAIDs, repairing intestinal tract damage and resolving inflammation, measuring and correcting cortisol imbalances, choosing to eat properly, and/or learning to understand what your opinions and judgments are and how deeply they affect your life, you **can** regain your health and have a complete strategy for managing stress successfully.

I've shown you how to evaluate different types of therapy for health problems that are in the structural part of the triangle of health that will help you eliminate the need for the over-use of NSAIDs. You have the 3R Program to Resolve inflammation, Repair the intestinal tract, and Restore hormonal balance. We've established the fundamentals of a healthy diet for the chemical side of the triangle. And lastly, you're armed with strategies to help you understand how your opinions and thought processes effect the emotional side of the triangle.

You now have a blueprint to regain and maintain vibrant health.

When I first decided to write this book, my purpose was to be able to take the procedures I use successfully on a daily basis in my practice and extend them to a larger audience. While it's enormously fulfilling to help people regain their health on an individual basis, it became increasingly apparent, and alarming, that there are millions of people suffering from the effects of cortisol imbalances. As we've seen, these people have no idea that intestinal tract and/or systemic inflammation may be the cause of their feeling so stressed out, nor are they aware of the many and frightening symptoms that can result from cortisol imbalance. At its most tragic endpoint, this ugly and often bewildering complex of symptoms can and does erode health and ruin lives.

It's my sincere hope that you'll use any or all the resources listed at the end of this book to help you find out what your own cortisol levels are and to resolve any imbalances that might be present in your triangle of health.

Richard Weinstein, D.C.

A Review of the 3R Program

<u>R</u>epair the intestinal tract:

- L-glutamine: 1,500 mg morning and night on an empty stomach for six to eight weeks; if good progress is made, you can drop to 1,500 mg just once a day as preventative maintenance thereafter.

- Psyllium or guar gum fiber at roughly 6 to 10 grams morning and night in either capsule or powdered form as directed on the supplement's label.

- Probiotics: as recommended on label.

- Curcumin: 650 mg two times a day (already a part of the <u>R</u>esolve aspect of the program, below) with food.

- Resveratrol: 200 mg three times a day with food.

- Optional: acetyl-l carnitine 500 mg and alpha lipoic acid 250 mg (for good glutathione levels), once a day with food.

- After 6-8 weeks of taking L-glutamine: begin oregano oil as directed on label with food if a Candida yeast problem exists.

<u>R</u>esolve inflammation:

- Omega-3 oils: 2,000 mg two times a day with food.

- Curcumin: 650 mg two times a day (which you're already taking in the <u>R</u>epair aspect of the program, above).

<u>R</u>estore hormone balance:

This can only be addressed accurately with an ASI or other hormone test. If you're not working with a doctor who can give you the specific Biotics or Apex supplements I use, you may safely try the following:

- Chromium: 200 mcg twice a day for blood sugar support with food.

- Ginseng, holy basil, rhodiola: 200 mg of each three times a day with food for adrenal gland support.

- Phosphatidylserine: 100 mg three times a day with food for pituitary/hypothalamus support.

- Vitamin D3: 2,000 IU a day with food.

- Multiple vitamin and mineral supplement: for a really good quality one, go to a vitamin store, as this will ensure that you will get the B vitamins, vitamin C, and the minerals your body needs to function properly. You can't always assume that you're getting everything you need out of the foods you're eating even with a good diet. Check the label to see how much chromium the supplement contains; if it has 200mcg or more, then you won't have to take extra chromium (indicated in the Repair aspect of the program, above).

The Maintenance 3R Program

Once you have regained your health you're going to want to keep it that way and not let yourself gradually relapse and have to start all over again.

As I mentioned in the preface of this book, we live in challenging times, besieged by environmental toxins, genetically modified foods, and a virtual sea of estrogen from all the plastics that surround us. In order to remain healthy, your best bet is to stay on a maintenance 3R Program, as follows

- L-glutamine: 1,500 mg once a day on an empty stomach.

- Curcumin: 650 mg once a day.

- Psyllium or guar gum fiber at roughly 6 to 10 grams morning and night in either capsule or powdered form as directed on the supplement's label.

- Resveratrol: 200 mg once a day.
- Vitamin D3: 1,000 mg once a day.
- Omega-3 oil: 1,000 mg morning and night.
- Multiple vitamin: as directed on label.

GLOSSARY

3-R Program: a comprehensive program that addresses the fundamental causes of many illnesses and hormonal imbalances by Repairing the intestinal tract, Resolving inflammation, and Restoring hormone balance.

Acetylcholine: a neurotransmitter chemical that is essential in being able to form memory in the hypothalamus of the brain.

Acetyl-l-carnitine: an amino acid compound that helps in the making of glutathione.

Adaptogenic: the ability to adapt back to normal function, or in the case of nutritional supplements, the ability to raise, lower, or leave a function or hormone level unchanged.

Adrenal fatigue: the inability of the adrenal glands to secrete the required amounts of hormones necessary for the body to function normally.

Adrenal dysfunction: less than adrenal fatigue, but still the inability to always secrete the proper amount of required hormones.

Aldosterone: the adrenal hormone that regulates the body's mineral content.

Alpha lipoic acid: an antioxidant found in every cell, and which helps turn glucose into energy; with acetyl-l-carnitine, it helps make glutathione.

Androgenic: any of the steroid hormones that maintain masculine characteristics.

Androstenedione: an adrenal gland hormone that is the replacement for estrogen when women reach menopause. The inability of the adrenal glands to secrete this will result in hot flashes.

Antioxidants: any substance that reduces oxidation usually caused by free radicals, and it is the process of oxidation that causes cells to dysfunction by losing electrons.

Arachidonic acid: while a normal component in the body, it is an inflammatory cytokine that can contribute to joint pain and exacerbate inflammation throughout the body. Foods that are high in arachidonic acid are shell fish, most red meat, and hydrogenated oils.

ASI/Adrenal Stress Index test: a saliva test that measures a person's cortisol levels four times throughout the day and also tests for insulin and progesterone levels, intestinal tract inflammation, and sensitivity to gluten.

Aspartame: an artificial sweetener used in over 6,000 products that are usually labeled as "sugar free" or "diet"; it is a neurotoxin that kills brain cells.

Atherosclerosis: the process in which plaques of fat or other debris accumulates inside an artery and blocks normal blood flow.

Autonomic nervous system: the branch of our nervous system that handles everything we don't need to think of, such as digestive, immune, cardiovascular, and kidney function as examples. It is divided into sympathetic (generally increases activity) and parasympathetic (generally lowers activity) branches.

Avascular: lacking a blood supply.

Bioflavonoids: are a group of antioxidants found in citrus, tea, red wine, and chocolate.

Brachial plexus: the collection of nerves from the lower neck that are the nerve supply to the shoulder region and the arms all the way down to the finger tips.

Bradykinin: while a normal chemical peptide in the body, elevated levels can act as an irritant and increase pain, especially in joints. Bradykinins occur in a poorly-balanced pH diet that is overly acidic.

Bromelain: a proteolytic enzyme, which means it circulates through the body and reduces inflammation, and is especially effective in lowering bradykinin levels. Its primarily source is from pineapples, but it can be bought as a supplement.

Candida albicans: a yeast normal to the body, but an overgrowth due to intestinal tract inflammation can cause cravings for sugar and blood sugar disorders, and further degrade the intestinal tract lining.

Cerebral spinal fluid: the serum-like fluid that circulates throughout the brain and spinal cord carrying all of the essential nutrients to these tissues.

Circadian rhythm: having a 24 hour cycle.

Coenzyme: a vitamin-like substance that assists in transporting chemicals and helps cells make energy.

Colitis: inflammation of the colon.

Cox – 1, 2, & 3: these are enzymes that protect the lining of the intestinal tract and are inhibited by non-steroidal anti-inflammatory drugs (NSAIDs) such as ibuprophen, Advil, aspirin, and Aleve, and can result in intestinal tract inflammation.

Cortisol: an adrenal gland hormone that acts as an anti-inflammatory agent but is also the fight-or-flight stress hormone.

Cortisone: a pharmaceutical manufactured version of cortisol used to reduce inflammation and swelling.

Chronic adrenal stress: the condition where the adrenal glands are overworked to secrete cortisol in response to prolonged periods of inflammation and/or stress.

Craniosacral: the relationship between the bones of the skull and the sacrum (tailbone) for the purpose of circulating cerebrospinal fluid which occurs while breathing.

Cross-referencing: when food sensitivities cross over into a similar category, such as a wheat sensitivity now becoming a rice, corn, or other grain sensitivity.

Curcumin: an extract of turmeric that is an anti-inflammatory agent.

Cysteine: an amino acid found in high protein foods that makes glutathione in combination with the amino acids glycine and glutamic acid.

Cytokines: are chemical mediators that trigger cellular responses for normal human function. However, there are a group of inflammatory cytokines that disrupt normal function when they are abnormally elevated from intestinal tract inflammation or systemic inflammation from a poor diet.

Dehydroepiandrosterone (DHEA): an adrenal gland hormone that helps make sex hormones, is important in bone density, and helps with blood sugar regulation.

Diabetes mellitus: a hereditary form of diabetes when the pancreas cells that make insulin don't function.

Diverticulitis: an inflammation of the diverticuli or pouches of the colon.

Dopamine: a neurotransmitter chemical in the brain that is associated with the pleasure response but is therefore also associated with addictions.

Endorphins: opiate chemicals produced in the brain.

Epinephrine: an adrenal gland hormone that is important for clarity of thought and keeping the bronchial tubes of the lungs open. Too little epinephrine can result in asthma and foggy thinking.

Estrogen: a hormone primarily associated with female hormone function but men also make estrogen from their adrenal glands whereas women make it from their ovaries.

Excitotoxins: primarily glutamate, which is part of monosodium glutamate (MSG) with the monosodium taken out, that is intentionally put in processed and fast foods to make them addictive. Aspartame is also an excitotoxin, and these substances actually excite (excito) the brain cells to a point of death (toxin).

Exercised induced asthma: this occurs when the demand for the adrenal glands to make cortisol is so high that they can't make adequate amounts of epinephrine and norepinephrine, which keep the bronchial tubes open, and asthma ensues as exercise increases the demand for cortisol.

Free Radical: an atom or a group of atoms with at least one unpaired (hence the term "free") electron that can cause disruption in the molecular balance of other atoms. On a cellular level it can cause abnormal function.

Fibromyalgia: an autoimmune disease where the immune system attacks muscle fibers.

Gastrin: a hormone released from the pituitary gland that instructs the stomach cells to secrete hydrochloric acid for digestion.

Glandular extracts: tissue from animal (usually cow, pig, and lamb) organs and glands used in nutritional supplements to support a similar human organ or gland. Such as adrenal extract to support adrenal gland function.

Glucogenesis: the process of cortisol breaking down muscle tissue and transporting it to the liver to make glucose (sugar) to feed the brain. This occurs when blood sugar levels drop below normal and is usually caused by a diet of insufficient protein intake.

Glucose: a form of sugar made from dietary carbohydrates that is created in the liver.

Glutamate: a protein amino acid that is derived from glutamine and is an excitatory neurotransmitter to the brain. Our body regulates how much glutamate is made from glutamine so there is no excess, but food manufacturers put it in their products because it is highly addictive, and causes cravings for that product. Glutamate is an excitotoxin that can kill brain cells.

Glutamine: a protein amino acid that is used by the body to repair the intestinal tract lining.

Glutathione: the most powerful antioxidant our body makes by combining three amino acids (glutamic acid, cysteine, and glycine) from the protein we eat. The amount of glutathione each of us makes is based on our genetic ability to do so, and can sometimes explain why a person with poor lifestyle habits can outlive a person with good lifestyle habits though the good luck of making more glutathione.

Gluten ataxia and gluten encephalopathy: both terms refer to an autoimmune attack on the brain caused by gluten found in wheat, oats, rye, and barley.

Gluteomorphine: a morphine made from today's hybridized (a form of genetic manipulation) gluten products. It explains why some people have serious cravings for bread and wheat products because they are making morphine in their brain from eating it and it is highly addictive.

Glycemic index: a list that shows the rate at which foods turn into sugar in the body. The higher the number, the more quickly sugar enters the blood stream. By example, whole grain bread is 72 and a Snickers bar is 41, so from a sugar standpoint which relates to weight gain and diabetes, the Snickers bar is far better!

H. Pylori: a bacteria that can infect the stomach and can cause digestive problems.

Hashimoto's thyroiditis: an autoimmune attack on the thyroid gland.

Histamine: is released by immune cells and initiates the inflammatory response most associated with allergies.

Homeostasis: the state of being in balance with physiological functions.

Hypoglycemia: low blood sugar caused by poor diet, not eating frequently enough, poor pancreatic function in secreting insulin, or elevated cortisol levels that are antagonistic to insulin.

Hypothalamus: the structure in the middle of the brain that perceives incoming information from our senses and is adjacent to the pituitary gland that regulates all hormone activity. It is where short-term memory is made and stored, and where emotional memory is processed and stored.

Hypothyroidism: low functioning of the thyroid gland resulting in symptoms that include fatigue, cold extremities, weight gain due to slow metabolism (the ability to burn calories properly), hair loss, and unclear or foggy thinking.

Inflammation: as used in this book, means the irritation if tissue, such as the lining of the intestinal tract, from a diet that is high in inflammatory omega 6 oils, poor diet, and the overuse of anti-inflammatory medications (aspirin, Advil, ibuprophen), and or antibiotics. It also refers to systemic inflammation which is the elevation of cytokines in the bloodstream due to a diet high in omega 6 oils.

Interleukins: there are twelve of these chemical messengers (neurotransmitters) that direct the function of the immune system. They are numbered as IL1, IL2, and so on.

Insulin-dependent diabetes: refers to diabetes mellitus where the pancreas cell don't secrete insulin and so the person is dependent on insulin medication.

Insulin resistance: the inability to use your own insulin to metabolize sugar due to elevated levels of cortisol, which is antagonistic to insulin. This will cause weight gain, diabetes, mood swings and irritability, and cravings for sugar.

Irritable bowel syndrome: a catch phrase for any number of causes for the digestive tract below the stomach to be inflamed.

L-tyrosine: the nutritional supplement variety of tyrosine, which is a protein amino acid critical in making thyroid hormone.

Lamina: referring to layers of a structure.

Leaky gut syndrome: this occurs when the lining of the intestinal tract has become so inflamed that microscopic holes develop and allows toxins, poorly digested bits of food, and microbes to leak out. This can trigger an immune response to the particles that leak out.

Leptin: a hormone that tells the brain when you've had enough to eat and also helps the body burn fat.

Leptin resistance: this is when leptin is not able to attach to the brain's receptor sites due to cortisol and blood sugar imbalances and the brain doesn't know when to send the signal to stop eating.

Lumbosacral plexus: these are the nerves exiting the lumbar or lower back vertebrae and sacrum (tailbone) that are the nerve supply of the lower limbs and organs in the reproductive tract, bladder, and lower intestinal tract.

Lupus: an autoimmune disease of the skin and mucous membranes.

Mechanoreceptors: these are nerve cells inside every joint in the body that tell the brain what position the joint is in and when under stimulated because the joint is not aligned properly, they turn on the pain nerves (nociceptors) so the brain knows that something is wrong.

Melatonin: a hormone from the pineal gland in the brain that has the opposite circadian rhythm of cortisol and is highest at night to make you sleepy.

Multiple sclerosis: an autoimmune attack on the protective myelin sheath of the nerves, often resulting in first numbness and then paralysis.

Neuro-emotional complexes: this when emotional events get locked into different parts of the body, such as the neck, lower back or adrenal glands, and become a vicious cycle of dysfunction. For example, a childhood abuse situation can get locked up with adrenal gland function, and anything that reminds you of the abuse triggers adrenal dysfunction. However, it is a two way street, in that chronic pain or illness can cause frustration over not getting well, yet every time you get frustrated, you perpetuate the pain or illness.

Neuro-Emotional Technique: this is a methodology developed by Scott Walker, D.C. that normalizes negative physical and/or behavioral patterns that have become locked up in the body.

Neurotransmitter/neuropeptide: interchangeable terms for a chemical substance released from nerve endings that transmits impulses to affect muscle, nerve, and organ activity.

Non-insulin dependent diabetes: diabetes caused either by the pancreas cells being worn out and unable to make insulin or elevated levels of cortisol that makes insulin unable to attach to receptor sites, known as insulin resistance.

Non-steroidal anti-inflammatory drugs (NSAIDs): a class of drugs that include aspirin, Advil, Aleve, Motrin, Celebrex, Anaprox, and Feldine used for pain and inflammation. The prolonged use of these drugs, typically thirty days or more, can cause inflammation of the intestinal tract lining because the block the cox enzymes that repair the intestinal tract.

Norepinephrine: an adrenal hormone that stimulates the sympathetic part of the nervous system, causes vasoconstriction (narrowing of the blood vessels), and acts as a neurotransmitter in the brain.

Omega 6 oils: while an essential fatty acid necessary for human function, elevated amounts cause inflammation that trigger a cortisol response. While a normal ratio of omega 6 oils to omega 3 oils should be 4 to 1, the average American diet is as high as 25 to 1 due to the consumption of fast food, processed food, and anything containing corn product (high fructose corn syrup and corn syrup) as corn is highly inflammatory.

Papain: an enzyme from papaya that reduces inflammation.

Pancreatin: a digestive enzyme secreted from the pancreas.

Pepsin: a digestive enzyme secreted from the stomach. (Papain, pancreatin, and pepsin are commonly found in nutritional supplements to aid digestion. They can also be taken on an empty stomach to reduce inflammation and are then called proteolytic enzymes.)

Phosphatidylserine: concentrated mainly in brain cells, it helps regulate hypothalamus and pituitary gland function.

Pituitary gland: often referred to as "the master gland", the pituitary controls the secretions of all of the other hormonal glands.

Pregnenalone: is the building block material from which all hormones are made, and it is primarily secreted by the adrenal glands.

Pregnenalone steal: this describes the adrenal glands having dominance over, or hogging up, the use of pregnenalone to make cortisol at the expense of other hormonal glands not being able to get enough to make their hormones.

Primary respiratory function: is the circulation of cerebral spinal fluid from the brain down through the spinal cord and back again that occurs with breathing.

Probiotic: a nutritional supplement that has numerous strains of beneficial bacteria that are essential for normal intestinal tract function.

Progesterone: a female hormone secreted by the ovaries to help prepare the uterus for implantation of a fertilized ovum (egg) and is also important in thyroid function.

Pro-inflammatory diet: a diet high in inflammatory omega six oils usually coming from fast food, processed food, corn, and wheat products.

Proprioception: refers to sensory nerve endings found in muscles and joints that maintain a sense of balance and coordination.

Prostaglandins: a variety of substances that can effect hormonal activity and are often involved in an inflammatory response.

Proteolytic enzymes: these are enzyme such as papain, pepsin, bromelain, and pancreatin that, when taken on an empty stomach, will breakdown inflammatory substances in the body, thus reducing pain and swelling of tissues.

Psoas muscle: this helps to attach the ball of the hip joint into the socket, then is firmly attached to all five lumbar (lower back) vertebra, and then finally ends by attaching to the last two vertebra of the shoulder girdle that have ribs. The two psoas muscles are in the front of the spine and when contracted one at a time they enable us to walk, run, climb stairs, and ride a bike. When they both contract, they enable us to bend over at the waist, or if lying down we can bring our knees up towards our chest. When they go into a spasm from lifting improperly, they are a major cause of lower back pain, and can also cause shoulder pain by pulling the shoulder girdle out of alignment.

Pycnogenol: an antioxidant that comes from maritime pine trees.

Receptor site: this is the docking structure on the outside of a cell wall that allows chemicals, nutrients, and hormones to get in and out of the cell.

Resveratrol: the extract from red grape skin that is a powerful anti-inflammatory agent.

Rheumatoid arthritis: an autoimmune disease that attacks the joints.

Sacral: refers to the sacrum or tailbone at the base of the spinal column.

Sacral occipital technique: a method of manually adjusting or moving the cranial bones of the skull to correspond with the breathing pattern that allows for the circulation of cerebral spinal fluid.

Self-tolerance: describes how the immune system recognizes the body's own tissues or cells and doesn't launch an immune attack on them.

Serotonin: a brain neurotransmitter that is responsible for the feeling of well-being.

SigA or Secretory IgA: an antibody that binds to harmful microorganisms to prevent them from damaging the intestinal tract lining.

Stage two detoxification: describes how the body gets rid of toxins in the bloodstream. All blood circulates back to the liver, which then screens out and breaks down toxins and waste material, including hormones. If the toxins are fat soluble, the liver ships them into the intestinal tract where they are excreted with the bowel movement. If the toxins are water soluble they are excreted by the kidneys through urination. In the case of leaky gut syndrome, the toxin leak out back into the bloodstream and continually circulate back to the liver, which puts a strain on liver function.

Sympathetic/parasympathetic nervous systems: see autonomic nervous system.

Systemic inflammation: the presence of inflammatory chemicals circulating in the bloodstream that will trigger an cortisol response to reduce the inflammation. This is caused by a pro-inflammatory diet of fast foods, processed foods, corn and wheat products, and even negative emotions that cause an increase in inflammatory cytokines.

T-cells: immune cells that arise from the thymus gland.

Testosterone: primarily a male hormone produced in the testicles that causes male dominant characteristics, but is also present in women and can influence sex drive.

Thymus gland: an immune gland located in the chest that produced T-cells that circulate throughout the body to kill invading microorganisms such as viruses and bacteria.

Thyroid gland: a hormonal gland located in the throat that secretes hormones that dictate the rate that calories are burned (metabolism), body temperature, mental alertness, and mood.

Unbound bioactive fraction: this is the actual state in which a hormone works and causes an effect in the body. This is what the Adrenal Stress Index (ASI) tests for whereas blood tests are only able to measure the amount of a hormone while it is still bound to a protein that is carrying the hormone to a receptor site. Until the hormone is "unbound" its usefulness is not realized.

Villi: these are finger-like projections in the intestinal tract that absorb nutrients.

Xenobiotics: these are a class of toxins from plastics, organic solvents, pesticides, and industrial wastes in water and air. Xeno indicates strange, foreign, or different. An example would be xenoestrogen, which comes from plastics and to the body, it looks just like estrogen and has the same effect that ovarian secreted estrogen has.

NO WONDER YOU FEEL LIKE CRAP!

RESOURCE GUIDE

Laboratories for Hormone Testing

Diagnos-Techs, Inc.
6620 192nd Place, Bldg. J, Kent, WA 98032 (425) 251-0596
e-mail: cs@diagnostechs.com

Genova Laboratory
63 Zillicon Street Asheville, NC 28801 (800) 522-4762

Meridian Valley Laboratory
515 West Harrison Street, Suite 9, Kent, WA 98032
(253) 859-8700

Cyrex Lab
5040 N. 15th Avenue, Suite 107, Phoenix, AZ, 85015
(602) 759-1245

Chiropractic Care and Specific Adjusting Techniques

American Chiropractic Association
1701 Claredon Blvd., Arlington, VA 22209
(800) 986-4636

International Chiropractic Association
1110 N. Glebe Road, Suite 1000, Arlington, VA 22201
(800) 423-4690

Richard Weinstein, D.C.

Activator Method: this chiropractic adjusting technique uses a handheld adjusting instrument that delivers a specific, light thrust to the joint being treated. It's very gentle, and there is no cracking or popping of the joints. To find a chiropractor near you who uses this method, call 800-598-0224.

Direct Non-Force Technique (DNFT): this method is also very gentle and adjusts the joints by using a quick thrust of the doctor's thumb on the joint being treated. To find a chiropractor near you who uses this technique, go to www.nonforce.com .

Sacro-Occipital Technique: this technique uses cushioned wedges specifically placed under the patient, allowing gravity to realign the lower back. The technique also adjusts joints in the more traditional manner of applying a quick thrust to the joints that causes a popping sound, and includes cranial adjusting. To find a chiropractor who uses this method, check the website www.sorsi.com or search the Internet for Chiropractic + Sacro Occipital Technique

Nutritional Supplements

D.S.D. International, Ltd.: Distributor of Biotics nutritional supplements in California, Arizona, and New Mexico. To find a doctor who is familiar with these supplements, call (800) 232-3183.

Biotics Research Corporation: The manufacturer of Biotics nutritional supplements; call (800) 231-5777.

Apex Energetics
(800) 736-4381

REFERENCES

Preface

Hyman, Mark, M.D., *Ultrametabolism*, Scribner, 2006, pg. 129

Seaman, David, R., The Diet Induced Proinflammatory State: A Cause of Chronic Pain and Other Degenerative Diseases, *Journal of Mainipulative and Physiological Therapeutics*, March 29, 2001.

Chapter 4: Testing Cortisol Levels

Baxendale, P. M.; and James, V. H. T. 1983. *Immunoassays for Clinical Chemistry*. New York: Churchill Livingstone, 430—44.

Berthonneau, J.; Tanguy, G.; Janssens, Y.; et al. 1989. *Human Reprod.* 4: 625-28.

Connor, M. L.; Sanford, L. M.; and Howland, B. E. 1982. *Can. J. Physiol. Pharmacol.* 60: 410-13.

Cook, N. J.; Read, G. F; Walker, R. F; Harris, B.; and Riad-Fahmy, D. 1986. *Eur. J. Appl. Physiol.* 55: 634-38.

DeBoever, J.; Kohen, F.; Bouve, J.; Leyseele, D.; and Vanderkerckhove, D. 1990. *Clin. Chem.* 36: 2036-41.

Evans, J. J.; Stewart, C. R.; and Merrick, A. Y. 1980. *Br. J. Obstet. Gynaecol.* 87: 624-26.

Ferguson, D. B. 1984. *Front. Oral. Physiol.* 5: 1-162.

Fischer-Rasmussen, W.; Gabrielsen, M. V.; and Wisborg, T. 1982. *Acta. Obstet. Gynecol.* 60: 417-20..

Frisch, R. E. 1987. *Hum. Reprod.* 2: 521-33.

Gaskell, S. J.; Pike, A. W.; and Griffiths, K. 1980. *Steriods.* 36: 219-28.

Gould, V. J.; Turkes, A. O.; and Gaskell, S.J. 1986. *J. Steriod Biochem.* 24: 563-67.

Guechot, J., et al. 1987. *Neuropsychobiology.* 18: 1—4.

Kahn, J. P.; Rubinow, D. R.; Davis, C. L.; Kling, M.; and Post, R. M. 1988. *Biol. Psychiatry.* 23: 335-49.

Laudat, M. H.; Cerdas, S.; Fourier, C.; and Guiban, D.; et al. 1988. *J. Clin. Endocrinol. Metab.* 66: 343-48.

Lipson, S. F., and Ellison, P. T. 1989. *Am. J. Human Biol.* 1: 249-55.

Malamud, D. 1992. *Br. Med. J.* 305: 207-8.

Mandel, I. D. 1993. *Ann. N.Y. Acad. Sci.* 694: 1-10.

Mandel, I. D. 1990 *Oral Pathol.* 19: 119-25.

Meulenberg, P. M" and Hoffinan, J. A. 1989. *Clin. Chem.* 35: 168-72.

Mounib, N.; Sultan, C. H.; Bringer, J.; Hedon, B.; Nicolas, J. C.; Cristol, P.; Bressot, N.; and Descomps. 1988. *J. Steroid Biochem.* 31: 861—65.

O'Connor, P.; and Corrigan, D. L. 1987. *Med. Sci. Sports Exercise.* 19: 224-28.

Peters, L. R.; Walker, R. F.; Riad-Fahmy, D.; and Hall, R. 1982. *Clin. Endocrinol.* 17: 583-92.

Ratcliffe, J. G. 1985. *Adrenal Cortex.* Eds. Anderson, D. C., and Winter, J. D. 188-205.

Read, G. F.; Harper, M. E.; Peeling, W. B.; and Griffiths, K. 1981. *Int. J. Androl.* 4: 623-21.

Robinson, J.; Walker, S.; Read, G. F.; and Riad-Fahmy, D. 1981. *Lancet.* 1111-12.

Smith, R. G.; Besch, P. K.; Dill, B.; and Buttram Jr., V. C. 1979. *Fertil. Steril.* 31: 513.

Tarui, H., and Nakamura, A. 1987. *Aviat. Space Environ Med..* 58: 573-75.

Tunn, S.; Mollmann, H.; Barth, J.; Derendorf, H.; and Kreig, M. 1992. Clin. Chem. 38: 1491-94. Turkes, A. O., and Read, G. F. 1984. *Immunoassays of Steriods in Saliva.* Cardiff: Alpha Omega, 228-38.

Umeda, T.; Hiramatsu, R.; Iwaoka, T.; Shimada, T.; Miura, F.; and Sato, T. 1981. *Clin. Chem. Acta..* 110: 245-53.

Vining, R. F.; McGinley, R. A.; Maksvytis, J. J.; and Ho, K. Y. 1983. *Ann. Clin. Biochem.* 20: 329-35.'

Vining, R. F.; McGinley, R. A.; and Symons, R. G. 1983. *Clin. Chem..* 29: 1752-56.

Vuorento, T.; Lahti, A.; Hovatta, O.; Huhtaniemi, I., 1989. *Scand. J. Clin. Lab. Invest..* 49: 395-401.

Walker, R., et al. 1982. Ninth Tenovus Workshop, Cardiff U.K.

Walker, R. F.; Wilson, D. W.; Read, G. F.; and Riad-Fahmy, D. 1980. *Int. J. Androl..* 3: 105.

Walker, S. M.; Walker, R. F.; and Riad-Fahmy, D. 1984. *Horm. Res..* 20: 231-40.

Wong, Y. F.; Mao, K.; Panesar, N.; Loong, E. P. L.; Chang, A. M. Z.; and Mi, Z.J. 1990. *Eur. J. Obstet. Gynecol. Reprod. Biol..* 34: 129-35.

Chapter 5: The Relationship of Cortisol to Other Diseases

Almy, T., 1951. "Experimental studies on irritable colon," *Amer. J. Med..* 10: 60.

Barnes, B. O., and Galton, L. 1976. *Hypothyroidism: the Unsuspected Illness..* New York: Harper & Row

Bird, C. E.; Masters, V.; and Clark, A. F. 1984. "Dehydroepiandrosterone sulfate: kinetics of metabolism in normal young men and women," *Clin. Invest. Med..* 7: 119—22.

Born, J., et al. 1991. "Gluco- and antimineralocorticoid effects on human sleep: a role of central corticosteroid receptors," *Amer. J. Physiol.*. E183—E188.

Born, J., et al. 1986. "Night-time plasma cortisol secretion is associated with specific sleep stages," *Bio. Psychiat.*. 21: 1415—24.

Buske-Kirschbaum, A.; Jobst, S.; Psych, D.; Wustmans, A.; Kirschbaum, C.; Rauh, W.; and Hellhammer, D. 1997. "Cortisol responses to psychosocial stress in children with atopic disorders," *Psychosomatic Med.*

Carroll, B. J., et al. 1981. "A specific laboratory for the diagnosis of melancholia," *Arch. Med. Psychiat.* 38: 15—22.

Carroll, B.J., et al. 1976. "Neuroendocrine regulation in depression," *Arch. Med. Psychiat.* 33: 1051-58.

Champe, P. C., and Harvey, R. A. 1992. *Lippincott Illustrated Reviews*. Biochemistry.

Cleary, M. P., and Zisk, J. F. 1986. "Anti-obesity effect of two different levels of dehydroepiandrosterone in lean and obese middle-aged female zucker rats," *Int. J. Obesity*. 10: 193-204.

Croes, M. P., et al. 1993. "Cortisol reaction in success and failure condition in endogenous depressed patients and controls," *Psyconeuroendocrin*. 18: 23-35.

Cutolo, M.; Balleari, E.; Giusti, M.; et al. 1991. "Androgen replacement therapy in male patients with rheumatoid arthritis," *Arthritis Rheum*. 34: 1—5.

DeMarco, VG, Johnson, MS, Whaley-Connell, AT, "Cytokine abnormalities in the etiology of the cardiometabolic syndrome", *Curr. Hypertens. Rep*, 2010 April; 12 (2); 93-8.

De Feo, P., et al. 1989. "Contribution of cortisol to glucose counterregulation in humans," *Amer. J. Physiol.* 257: E35—E42.

Demitrack, M. A., et al. 1991. "Evidence for impaired activation of the hypothalamic-pituitary-adrenal axis in patients with chronic fatigue syndrome," *J. Clin. Endocrin. Metab.*. 73: 1224-34.

Desiderado, O.; MacKinnon, J.; and Hissom, R. 1974. "Development of gastric ulcers following stress termination," *J. Comp. and Physiol. Psych.* 87: 208.

Dey, A. C., et al. 1972. "Excretion of conjugated ll-deOxy-17-ketosteriods in 'Essential' hypertension", *Can. J. Biochem.* 50: 1273-81.

Donald, R. A., et al. 1994. Plasma corticotrophin releasing hormone, vasopressin, ACT H and Cortisol responses to acute myocardial infarction," *Clin. Endocrin.* 40: 499-504.

Feldman, M.; Walker, P.; Green, J.; and Weingarden, K. 1986. "Life events, stress and psychosocial factors in men with peptic ulcer disease: a multidimensional case-controlled study," *Gastroenterol.* 91: 1370.

Foldes, J., et al. 1983. "Dehydroepiandrosterone sulfate (DS), dehydroepiandrosterone (D), and 'free' dehydroepiandrosterone (FD) in the plasma with thyroid diseases," *Horm. Metab. Res.* 15: 623—24.

Freiss, E.; Trachsel, L.; Guldner, J.; Schier, T.-; Steiger, A.; and Holsboer, F. 1995. "DHEA administration increases rapid eye movement sleep and EEG power in the sigma frequency range," *Am. J. of Physiol.* 268 (Endorcrin Metab. 31): E107-E113.

Gansler, T.; Meller, S.; and Cleary, J., 1985. "Chronic administration of dehydroepiandrosterone reduces pancreatic B-cell hyperplasia and hyperinsulinemia in genetically obese zucker rats," *Pro. Soc. Exp. Biol. Med.* 180: 155-62.

Gheorghiu, T., and Hubner, G. 1975. "Morphological and functional gastric changes in stress ulcer," *Experimental Ulcer: Models, Methods, and Clinical Validity.* Baden-Baden: Witzstrock.

Hall, G. M.; Perry, L. A.; and Spector, T. D. 1993. "Depressed levels of dehydroepiandrosterone sulfate in postmenstrual women with rheumatoid arthritis but no relation with axial bone density," *Am. Rheum.* 52: 211—14.

Hedman, M.; Nilsson, E.; and de la Torre, B. 1989. "Low sulpho-conjugated steroid hormone levels in systemic lupus erythematosus," *Clin. Exp. Rheumatol.*. 7: 583-88.

Heimke, C., et al, 1994. "Circadian variations in antigen-specific proliferation of human T lymphocytes and correlation to cortisol production," *Psychoneuroendocrin.* 20: 335—42.

Holmes, G. P., et al. 1987. "A cluster of patients with a chronic mononucleosis-like syndrome: Is Epstein-Barr virus the cause? *JAMA.* 257: 2297— 2302.

Hong Din, J. U., et al. 1988. "High serum cortisol levels in exercise associated amenorrhea," *Ann. Int. Med.* 108: 530-34.

Kaplan, J. "Social behavior and gender in biomedical investigations using monkeys: Studies in atherogenesis," *Laboratory Animal Science.*

Kumar, D., and Wingate, D. 1988. "Irritable bowel syndrome," *An Illustrated Guide to Gastrointestinal Motiltiy*. Chichester: John Wiley.

Manolagas, S. C., et al. 1979. "Adrenal steroids and the development of osteoporosis in the oophorectomized women," *Lancet.* 2: 597.

Marin, P., et al. 1992. "Cortisol secretion in relation to body fat distribution in obese menopausal women," *Metab.* 41: 882—86.

Meikle, A. W, et al. 1992. "The presence of dehydroepiandrosterone-specific receptor binding complex in murine T cells," *Am J. Med. Sci.* 303: 366—71.

Miller, J. E., et al. 1994. "Characterization of 24 hour cortisol release in obese and non-obese hyperandrogenic women," *Gynecol. Endocrin.* 8: 247—54.

Murison, R., and Bakke, H. 1990. "The role of corticotrophin-releasing factor in rat gastric ulcerogenesis," *Neurobiology of Stress Ulcers.* Annals of the New York Academy of Sciences, vol. 597.

Nordin, B. E. C., et al. 1985. "The relation between calcium absorption, serum dehydroepiandrosterone, and vertebral mineral density in post-menopausal women," *J. Clinic. Endocrin. Metab.* 60: 651-57.

Nowaczynski, W., et al.1967. "Further evidence of altered adrenocortical function in hypertension. Dehydroepiandrosterone excretion rate," *Can. J. Biochem.* 46: 1031-38.

Opstad, K. 1994. "Circadian rhythm of hormones is extinguished during prolonged physical stress, sleep and energy deficiency in young men," *Eur. J. Endocrin.* 131: 56—66.

Reaven, G.; Bernstein, R.; Davis, B.; and Olefski, J. 1976. "Nonketotic diabetes mellitus: Insulin deficiency or insulin resistance?" *Amer. J. Med.*

Sachar, E. J., et al. 1973. "Disrupted 24 hour patterns of cortisol secretion in depressive illness," *Arch. Gen. Psychiat.* 28: 19—24.

Schuster, M. 1989. "Mucus secretion decreases with stress and glucocorticoid administration." In Sleisenger, M., and Fordtron, J. *Gastrointestinal Disease: Pathophysiology, Diagnosis, Management*, 4th ed. Philadelphia: Saunders.

Stahl, H., et al. 1992. "Dehydroepiandrosterone levels in patients with pro-static cancer, heart diseases, and under surgery stress," *Exp. Clin. Endocrin.* 99: 68-70.

Straus, S., et al. 1998. *J. Allergy and Clin. Immunol.* 81: 79.

Suzuki, T.; Suzuki, N.; Engleman, E. G.; Mizushima, Y.; and Sakane, T. 1995. "Low serum levels of dehydroepiandrosterone may cause deficient IL-2 production by lymphocytes in patients with systemic lupus erythematosus," *Clin. Exp. Immunol.* 99: 251—55.

Thompson, D.; Richelson, E.; and Malagelada, J. 1982. "Perturbation of gastric emptying and duodenal motility through the central nervous system," *Gastroenterol.* 83: 1200.

Von Zerssen, D., et al. 1987. "Diurnal variation of mood and the cortisol rhythm in depression and normal states of mind," *Eur. Arch. Psychiat. Neurol. Sci.* 237: 36-45. Williams, Janice, Circulation. Chapel Hill: University of North Carolina.

Williams, Janice, *Circulation*, Chapel Hill: University of North Carolina .

Chapter 6: Resolving Cortisol Imbalances

Akgul, A., and Kivane, M. 1988. "Inhibitory effects of selected Turkish spices and oregano components on some food-borne fungi," *Int. J. Food Microbiology.* 6: 263.

Alverdy, J. A. 1990. "The effect of total parenteral nutrition in gut lamina propria cells," *J. Parent Enteral Nutr.* 14 (suppl.).

Conner, D. E., and Beuchat, L. D. 1984. "Effects of essential oils from plants on growth of food spoilage yeasts," *J. Food Science.* 49: 429.

Deighton, N.; Glidewell, S. M.; Deans, S. G.; and Goodman, B. A. 1933. "Identification by EPR spectroscopy of carvacrol and thymol as the major sources of free radicals in the oxidation of plant essential oils," *J. Science Food Agriculture.* 63: 221.

Fox, A. D., et al. 1988. "Effects of glutamine-supplemented enteral diet on methotrexate-induced enterocolitis," *JPEN.* 12: 325—31.

Fuert; S., and Fox, L. "Effects of orally administrating Spanish moss," *Science.* 1053: 626-27.

Gardner, M. L. G. 1988. "Gastrointestinal absorption of intact proteins," *Annu. Rev. Nutrition.* 8: 329-50.

Gardner, M. L. G. 1984. "Intestinal assimilation of intact peptides and proteins from the diet, a neglected field," *Biol. Rev.* 59: 289-331.

Genova, R., and Guerra, A. 1988. "A thymomodulin management of food allergy," *Int. J. Tiss. React.* 8: 239-42.

Gibson, G. R., et al. 1995. "Dietary modification of the human microbiota: introducing the concept of prebiotics," *J. Nutrition.* 125: 1401—12.

Haigler, E. D. 1972. "Response to orally administered synthetic thyrotropinreleasing hormone in man," *J. Clin. Endocrin. Metab.* 631—35.

Hidaka, H., et al. '1990. "The effects of undigestible fructooligosaccharides on intestinal microflora and various physiological functions on human health," *New Developments in Dietary Fiber*. New York: Plenum Press. 105-117.

Huang, K. F. 1983. "Study of the absorption of peptide from thymus extract when administered orally," *Erfahrungs-Heilkunde*. Bd32, H. 11.

Iantomai, T., et al. 1994. "Glutathione metabolism in Crohn's disease," *Biochem. Med. Metab. Biol.* 53: 87-91.

Julius, M., et al. 1994. "Glutathione and morbidity in a community-based sample of elderly," *J. Clin. Epedemiol.* 47: 1021—26.

Kumar, U. 1996. "Purification and characterization of chromogranin-A from the adrenal glands of human and bovine donors," *Biochem. Mol. Biol. Int.* 40: 83-91.

Lin, C-Y., and Low, T. L. K. 1989. "A comparative study of the immunological effects of bovine and porcine thymic extracts: induction of lymphoproliferative responses and enhancement of interleukin-2, interferon and tumor necrotic factor production in vitro on cord blood lymphocytes," *Immuno. Pharacol.* 18: 1—10.

Lin, C-Y., et al. 1987. "Treatment of combined immunodeficiency with thymic extract," *Annals. Allergy.* 58: 379-84:

Miller, J. M., and Ophershaw. 1964. "The increased proteolytic activity of human blood serum after the oral administration of bromelain," *Exp. Med. Surg.* 22: 277-80.

Monteleone, P.; Maj, M.; Beinat, L.; Natale, M.; and Kemali, D. 1992. "Blunting by chronic phosphatidylserine administration of the stress-induced activation of the hypothalamo-pituitary-adrenal axis in healthy men," *European J. Clin. Pharmacol.* 42(4): 385-88.

Monteleone, P.; Maj, M.; Beinat, L.; Tanzillo, C.; and Kemali, D. 1990. "Effects of phosphatidylserine on the neuroendocrine response to physical stress in humans," *Neuroendocrinol.* 52(3): 243—58.

Morton, J. F. *Atlas of Medicinal Plants of Middle America.* Springfield, 111.: Charles C. Thomas.

Murch, S. H., et al. 1993. "Disruption of sulfated glycosaminoglycan in intestinal inflammation," *Lancet.* 341: 711-14.

Okabe, S.; Takeuchi, K.; Honda, K.; and Takagi, K. 1976. "Effects of acetylsalicylic acid (ASA), ASA plus L-glutamine and L-glutamine on healing of chronic gastric ulcer in the rat," *Digestion.* 14: 85—88.

Oota, K., et al. 1976. "Clinical studies of Hi-Z pills on indefinite complaints of gastrointestinal neurosis, Yakuri to Chiryo," 4: 113. -

Sezik, E.; Tumen, G.; et al. 1933. "Essential oil composition of four origanum vulgare subspecies of Anatolian origin," J. Essent. Oil Res. 5: 425—31. Souba, W. W.; Smith, R. J.; and Wilmore, D. W. 1985. "Glutamine metabolism by the intestinal tract," *JPEN* 9: 608-17.

Steffen, C., et al. 1979. "Untersuchungen iiber intestinale Resorption mit 3H-markiertem, Enzymgemisch," *Acta. Med. Aust.* 6: 13—18.

Stein, J. 1967. "Objective demonstration of the organ-specific effectiveness of cellular preparations." In Schmidt, F., ed. *Cell Research and Cellular Therapy.* Ott Publishers. 294-301.

Svensen, A. B.; and Scheffer, J.J. C. 1985. *Essential Oils and Aromatic Plants.* Martinus Nijoff/W. Junk Publishers.

Vidaly Plama, R. R., et al. 1978. "Articular cartilage pharmacology: In vitro studies of glucosamine and nonsteroidal inflammatory drugs," *Pharm. Res. Commun.* 10: 557-69.

Wilmore, W. D. 1992. "The effect of glutamine on the gastrointestinal tract," *Rivista Ital. di Nutrz. Parent ed Enter.* 10: 1—6.

Wilson, J. L. 1996. "The anti-aging effects of liquid thymus extracts." In Klatz, R. ed. *Advances in Anti-Aging Medicine.* Vol. 1, 349—55.

Windmueller, H. G. 1982. "Glutamine Utilization by the Small Intestine," *Adv. Enzymol.* 53. 201-37.

Winslet, M. C., et al. 1994. "Mucosal glucosamine synthetase activity in inflammatory bowel disease," *Dig. Disease Sci.* 39: 540—44.

Yagi, Ohishi. 1976. "Action of ferulic acid and its derivatives as antioxidants," *J. Nutri. Sci. Vitaminol.* 206: 127.

Yokahama, S. 1984. "Intestinal absorption mechanisms of thyrotropinreleasing hormone," *J. Pharm. Dyn.* 7: 445—51.

Yoshimura, K., et al. 1993. "Effect of enteral glutamine administration on experimental inflammatory bowel disease," *JPEN.* 17: 235.

Zaloga, G. P. 1994. *Nutrition in Critical Care.* Mosby. 552-53.

Chapter 7: Make the Pain Go Away

Dean, D. H., and Schmidt, R. M. 1992. "A comparison of the costs of chiropractors versus alternative medical practitioners." Richmond, Virginia: University of Richmond.

Demographic Characteristics of Users of Chiropractic Services. 1991. The Gallup Organization. Princeton, New Jersey.

Ebrall, P. S. June 1992. "Mechanical low-back pain: a comparison of medical and chiropractic management within the Victorian work care scheme," *Chiropractic J. Australia.* 22 (2): 47-53.

Evidence Report: Behavioral and Physical Treatments for Tension-Type and Cervicogenic Headaches. May 2000. Duke University, Evidence-based Practice Center.

Hayek, Ray. 2002. *Advance.* 23: 2, 4..

Jarvis, K. B.; Phillips, R. B.; et al. August 1991. "Cost per case comparison of back injury claims of chiropractic versus medical management for conditions with identical diagnostic codes," *J. Occupational Med.* 33 (8): 847-52

Kandel, Eric. 2000. *Principals of Neural Science.* 482-85.

Ketsroser, D. B. February 2002. *Minnesota Medicine.* 83: 51-54.

Koes, B. W.; Bouter, L. M.; et al. 1992. "Randomized clinical trial of manipulative therapy and physiotherapy for persistent back and neck complaints: results of one year follow up," *Brit. Med. J.* 304: 601—5.

Linnman, Clas, April 6, 2011, "Elevated (11 C) D-Deprenyl Uptake in Chronic Whiplash Associated Disorder Persisten Musculoskeletal Inflammation", *Public Library of Medicine,* Vol. 6 No. 4, pp. e19182

MacDonald, M.J., and Morton, L.January 1986. "Chiropractic evaluation study task III report of the relevant literature," MRI Project No. 8533-D, for Department of Defense. OCHAMPUS. Aurora, Colorado.

Mayer, D.; Price, D.; Barber, J.; and Rafi, A. 1976. "Acupuncture analgesia: evidence for activation of a pain inhibitory system as a mechanism of action," *Advances in Pain Research and Therapy.* 1: 751.

Meade, T. W.; Dyer, S., et al. 1990. "Low back pain of mechanical origin: randomized comparison of chiropractic and hospital outpatient treatment," *Brit. Med. J.* 300 (67137): 1431-37.

Shekelle, P. G.; Adams, A.; et al. 1992. "The appropriateness of spinal manipulation for lower-back pain," Santa Monica, Calif.: RAND Corporation.

Steward, Oswald. 2000. *Functional Neuroscien.* New York: Springer. 218—19.

Wiberg, J. M. N.; Nordsteen, J.; and Nilsson, N. 1988. "The short-term effect of spinal manipulation in the treatment of infantile colic: a randomized controlled trial with a blinder observer," *J. Manip. Physiol. Ther.* 199: 22(8): 517-22; Klougart, N.; Nilsson, N.; and Jacobsen, J. 1989. "Infantile colic treated by chiropractors: a prospective study of 316 cases "*J. Manip. Physiol. Ther.* 12: 281-88; Lucassen, P. L.; Assendelft, W. J.; et al. 1988. "Effectiveness of treatments for infantile colic: systemic review" (published erratum appears in *BMJ.* 31 [7152]:171), BMJ. 316(7144): 1563-69; Adams, L. M., and Davidson, M. 1997. "Present concepts of infantile colic," *Pediatr. Ann.* 16: 817-20; Hide, D. W, and Guyer, B. M. 1983. "Prevalence of infantile colic," *Arch. Dis. Child.* 57(7): 559-60.

Wolk, S. September 1988. "Chiropractic versus medical care: a cost analysis of disability and treatment for back-related workers' compensation cases," Arlington, Virginia: Foundation for Chiropractic Education and Research.

Woodward, M. J.; Cook, et al. 1996. "Chiropractic treatment of chronic whiplash," *Injury.* 27(9): 643-45.

Chapter 8: The Not-So-Common Commonsense Diet

Barberger-Gateau, P.; Letenneur, L.; Deschamps, V.; Peres, K.; Dartigues, J-F.; and Renaud, S. October 26, 2002. "Fish, meat, and risk of dementia: a cohort study," *Brit Med. J.* 325: 932-33.

Hu, F. B., and Willet, W. C. November 27, 2002. "Optimal diets for prevention of coronary disease," *JAMA.* 288: 2569-78.

Miyamoto, H.; Saura, R.; Doita, M.; Kurasaka, M.; and Mizuno, K. November 15, 2002. "The role of cyclooxygenase-2 in lumbar disc herniation," *Spine.* 27(22): 2477-83.

Murray, M. July/August 1995. "GLA vs. omega-3 fatty acids in rheumatoid arthritis," *Amer. J. Nat. Med.* 2: 9-11.

Peet, M.; Glen, I.; and Horrobin, D. 2000. *Phospholipid Spectrum Disorder in Psychiatry.* Marius Press.

San Jose Mercury News. January 11, 2003, p. 2.

Schlosser, E. 2000. *Fast Food Nation.* Boston: Houghton Mifflin.

Chapter 10: The Emotional Component of Illness

Basmajian, J. V. 1989. *Biofeedback, Principals and Practice for Clinicicans.* 3rd. ed. Baltimore, MD: Williams & Wilkins.

Bohannon, R. 1997. "Internal consistency of manual muscle testing scores," *Perceptual and Motor Skills.* 85: 736-38.

Bohannon, R. 1997. "Reference values for extremity muscle strength obtained by hand-held dynaniometry from adults ages 20 to 70," *Arch. Phys. Med. and Rehab.* 78: 26-32.

Bonnet, M.; Bradley, M. M.; Lang, P. J.; and Requin, J. 1995. "Modulation of spinal reflexes; arousal, pleasure, and action," *Psycophysiol.* 32: 367—72.

Bradley, M. M.; Cuthbert, B. N.; and Lang, P.J. 1996. "Picture media and emotions: effects of a sustained affective context," *Psychophysiol.* 33: 662-70.

Bradley, M. T., and Cullen, M. C. 1993. "Polygraph lie detection on real events in a laboratory setting," *Perceptual and Motor Skills.* 76: 1051—58.

Burton, D. 1988. "Do anxious swimmers swim slower? Reexamining the elusive anxiety-performance relationship," *J. Sports and Exercise Psych.* 10: 45-61.

Cacioppo, J. T.; Uchino, B. N.; Crites, S. L.; Snydersmith, M. A.; Smith, G.; Bernstein, G. G.; and Lang, P.J. 1992. "Relationship between facial expressiveness and sympathetic activation in emotion: a critical review, with emphasis on modeling underlying mechanisms and individual differences," *J. Personality and Social Psych.* 62: 110—128.

Coren, S. 1993. "Measurement of handedness via self-report: the relationship between brief and extended inventories," *Perceptual and Motor Skills.* 76: 1035-42.

De Melo, F., and Laurent, M. 1996. "Effects of competitive activation on precision movement control," *Perceptual and Motor Skills.* 83: 1203—8.

Fischler, I.; Achariyapaopan, T.; and Perry, N. W. 1985. "Brain potentials during sentence verification: automatic aspects of comprehension," *Biol. Psych.* 23: 81-106.

Goodheart, G. 1964. *Applied Kinesiology.* Detroit, MI: private printing.

Gould, D.; Jackson, S.; and Finch, L. 1993. "Sources of stress in national figure skaters," *J. Sport and Exercise Physiol.* 15: 134—59.

Hsieh, C-Y., and Phillips, R. B. 1990. "Reliability of manual muscle testing with a computerized dynamometer," *J. Manip. and Physiol. Therapeutics.* 13: 72-82.

Lawson, A., and Calderon, L. 1997. "Interexaminer agreement for applied kinesiology manual muscle testing," *Perceptual and Motor Skills.* 84: 539—46.

Leisman, G.; Aenhausern, R.; Ferentz, A.; Terfer, T.; and Zemcov, A. 1995. "Electromyographic effects of fatigue and task repetition on the validity of strong and weak muscle estimates in Applied Kinesiological muscle testing," *Perceptual and Motor Skills.* 80: 933-46.

Levinson, R. W.; Ekman, P.; and Friesen, V. W. 1990. "Voluntary facial action emotion-specific autonomic nervous system activity," *Psychphysiol.* 27: 363-84.

Pennebaker, J. W.; Hughes, C. F.; and O'Heeron, R. C. 1987. "The psychophysiology of confession: linking inhibitory and psychosomatic processes," *J. Personality and Social Psych.* 52: 781—93:

Peterson, K. B. 1997. "The effects of spinal manipulation on the intensity of emotional arousal in phobic subjects exposed to threat stimulus: a randomized, controlled, double-blind clinical trial," *J. Manip. and Physiol. Therapeutics.* 20: 602—6.

Walker, S. 1992. "Ivan Pavlov, his dog, and chiropractic," *the Digest of Chiropractic Economics.* 34: 36—46.

Walker, S. 1996. *Neuro Emotional Technique: N.E.T. Basic Manual.* Encinitas, Calif. N.E.T. Inc.

Walther, D. S. 1990. *Applied Kinesiology. Vol. 1: Basic procedures and muscle testing.* Pueblo, Colo.: Systems, D.C.

Richard Weinstein, D.C.

ABOUT THE AUTHOR

Dr. Richard A. Weinstein has helped hundreds of patients with adrenal gland and other hormone imbalances, intestinal tract inflammation, leaky gut syndrome, Candida infections, and a host of other health disorders. As a chiropractor, he has been in private practice in Capitola, California, for thirty-five years.

A 1976 graduate of the New York Chiropractic College, he is a member of the *American Chiropractic Association* and its Council on Nutrition; the *National Institute of Chiropractic Research;* the *Foundation for Chiropractic Education and Research;* and the *California Chiropractic Association.*

In 1995 and 1996, Dr. Weinstein received the Botterman Award from the *California Chiropractic Association* for outstanding and dedicated service on behalf of the chiropractic profession.

DR. WEINSTEIN ONLINE

Please visit Dr. Weinstein's website at www.richardweinsteindc.com for updated information regarding cortisol and hormone research, as well as new strategies for regaining and maintaining vibrant health.

Reader support and word-of-mouth is vital for independent publishers and authors. If you enjoyed this book, please help spread the word by telling friends, mentioning it on social media, or posting a review online. Thank you so much.

NO WONDER YOU FEEL LIKE CRAP!

CPSIA information can be obtained
at www.ICGtesting.com
Printed in the USA
FSOW03n0908270417
33613FS